Disease and Social Diversity

Disease and Social Diversity

Disease and Social Diversity

The European Impact on the Health of Non-Europeans

Stephen J. Kunitz

Professor, Department of Community
and Preventive Medicine
University of Rochester
School of Medicine and Dentistry

New York   Oxford
OXFORD UNIVERSITY PRESS

Oxford University Press

Oxford New York
Athens Auckland Bangkok Bombay
Calcutta Cape Town Dar es Salaam
Delhi Florence Hong Kong Istanbul
Karachi Kuala Lumpur Madras Madrid
Melbourne Mexico City Nairobi Paris
Singapore Taipei Tokyo Toronto

and associated companies in
Berlin Ibadan

Copyright © 1994 by Oxford University Press, Inc.
First issued as an Oxford University Press paperback, 1996

Published by Oxford University Press Inc.,
198 Madison Avenue, New York, New York 10016

Library of Congress Cataloging-in-Publication Data
Kunitz. Stephen J.
Disease and social diversity :
the European impact on the health of non-Europeans /
Stephen J. Kunitz.
p. cm. Includes bibliographical references and index.
ISBN 0-19-508530-2 (cl) ISBN 0-19-510869-8 (pbk)
1. Epidemiology—Oceania—History.
2. Epidemiology—North America—History.
3. Indigenous peoples—Oceania—Health and hygiene.
4. Indigenous peoples—North America—Health and hygiene.
5. First contact of aboriginal peoples with Westerners—Oceania—Health aspects.
6. First contact of aboriginal peoples with Westerners—North America—Health aspects.
7. Cross-cultural studies.
I. Title.
[DNLM: 1. Disease Outbreaks—North America.
2. Disease Outbreaks—Pacific Islands.
3. Cross-Cultural Comparison.
WA 11 DA2 Kad 1994]
RA650.9.03K86 1994 614.4'295—dc20 93-35498

9 8 7 6 5 4 3 2 1

Printed in the United States of America
on acid-free paper

*This book is dedicated with love and admiration
to the memory of my parents,
Rae Bunim Kunitz and Joshua Kunitz.*

"There is no misfortune, but to act nobly is good fortune"
Marcus Aurelius

Preface

This book is about some of the many ways in which diverse social institutions and cultures shape patterns of disease and death in populations. My fascination with social diversity long preceded my interest in morbidity and mortality. In July 1965, having finished medical school and a year's training in internal medicine, I arrived with my hugely pregnant wife in Tuba City, Arizona, where we spent the next two years. My job was as a medical officer responsible for the extramural community programs provided by the Indian Health Service hospital, serving both Navajo and Hopi Indians. I have continued to do research in the Southwest off and on ever since. In providing health services and then becoming involved in social and epidemiologic research, I was struck by the differences between these two peoples who lived as neighbors in the same environment, and how those differences affected a variety of health-related measures.

Since then I have had the opportunity to work in several other places, including the former Yugoslavia and Oceania. Some of that work appears in this book, as does much of the work I have done in the American Southwest. What impressed me everywhere was how peoples' cultural values, social organization, patterns of subsistence, and political institutions all seemed to be importantly related to the health of the populations, but not in ways that were easily understandable, or necessarily generalizable from one place to another. Indeed, depending on the disease conditions of interest, different social variables seemed to be important.

This is a different view from that which writers on this topic usually take. Most of the time the contact between Europeans and non-Europeans in the Americas and Oceania is pictured as resulting in uniform population collapse of the latter following the introduction of new diseases by the former. Similarly, in more recent times declining rates of mortality and increasing rates of noninfectious diseases are described as part of a more or less uniform epidemiologic and demographic transition. While I do not deny either the horrific impact that epidemic diseases had on virgin soil populations, or the improvements that have taken place in the present century, I argue that too often the mediating role of social and political institutions and cultural values has not been taken sufficiently into account. My book is an attempt to redress the balance.

The problem that troubled me for a long time was how to write a coherent, integrated book about the story of diversity that I had observed and found to contribute significantly to disease patterns in the various places where I have worked. After all, if one is proposing a unifying theory, then theme and structure cohere. That was not my situation. I was trying to write a book which argued that many factors shape patterns of disease and death, and that their importance was determined largely by the outcome one was measuring. I finally settled on a series of comparative studies at increasingly refined levels of analysis in order to illustrate the many ways in which social institutions and cultural values influence disease patterns.

In many ways this is a deeply personal book. The examples are chosen because I have worked in certain places and not others. And why I got to many of these places was largely serendipitous. Other investigators might have gone elsewhere and chosen other examples to make not simply different but contradictory points. That is why I have written the book in the first person, and in the active rather than the passive voice. Scientific writing is generally impersonal and passive so as to create a sense of objectivity and omniscience. I believe that what I have written is in fact true; otherwise I would not have committed myself to print. But I am also acutely aware that the omniscient eye may be instead the all too fallible "I."

Rochester, N.Y.   S.J.K.
December 1993

Acknowledgments

So there I was, going about my business as usual, doing what I had always done, when out of the blue I was invited to spend three months a year for four years in Australia, at the National Centre for Epidemiology and Population Health at the Austrialian National University. It seemed like too interesting an opportunity to refuse. If nothing else, it would allow me to convince myself that Australia really existed, something about which I must confess I had had occasional doubts. My colleagues in the Department of Community and Preventive Medicine at the University of Rochester were embarrassingly and touchingly enthusiastic about the offer as well, even volunteering to pay the outward bound fare. With such encouragement and inducements, I could scarcely refuse.

The experience has been worth the long flights and absences from home during dreary Rochester winters, for it is a rare privilege to be given in middle age the opportunity that I have had. It has also been fun. Most of this book is the result of that opportunity, and my first debt of gratitude must therfore be to Bob Douglas and Jack Caldwell, the respective director and associate director of the National Centre for Epidemiology and Population Health, who extended the invitation and provided support.

Many other people in Australia have provided encouragement, advice, and assistance in the preparation of this book. It is a pleasure to acknowledge the help of Michael Bracher, Maggie Brady, Donald Denoon, Alan Gray, Bob Hogg, Ken Inglis, David Martin, Ian Ring, Claire Runciman, Gigi Santow, Barry Smith, Ric Streatfield, Peter Sutton, and Neil Thomson.

Chapter 2 is based on an article first published as "Public Policy and Mortality Among Indigenous Populations of Northern America and Australasia," in *Population and Development Review* 16 (December 1990):647–72. It is reprinted and modified with the permission of the Population Council.

Chapter 3 is a modified version of a chapter first published in C. G. Nicholas Mascie-Taylor, ed., *The Anthropology of Disease* (New York: Oxford University Press, 1993). It is used here with permission.

Chapters 5 and 6 are based on fieldwork in the American Southwest carried out in collaboration with my longtime colleague, Jerrold E. Levy. I am grateful to him for writing these chapters with me.

Finally, I am especially grateful to my wife Izzie for her encouragement of my work and her fortitude in my absences. She allowed herself to show only the slightest flicker of skepticism when I insisted it was crucial to the completion of this book, as well as for the advancement of learning, that I spend six weeks in Samoa, Tonga, and Tahiti, and several more considering at first hand the population history of the Great Barrier Reef.

Contents

Disease and Social Diversity

Disease and Social Diversity

1

Natural History and Local History

> Men that undertake only one district are much more likely to
> advance natural knowledge than those that grasp at more than
> they can possibly be acquainted with: every kingdom, every
> province, should have its own monographer.
>
> GILBERT WHITE

In a volume on the idea of social change and development in Western history, Robert Nisbet devotes considerable attention to the 18th-century idea of natural history:

> The method was to cut through the morass of customs, superstitions, traditions, and prescriptive laws, which to most of the rationalists of the age seemed to be the very stuff of the historic social order, to the underlying forces of the natural order. What was wanted was a conception of man's advancement through the ages in the terms of what was fundamental and natural to man, rather than in terms of ordinary or conventional history.[1]

The idea of nature, he continues, means pristine and "uncorrupted by adventitious circumstances. To get to the nature of anything is to get to its shape and substance before these have been altered by exposure to elements and forces not bound up in its own being."[2]

Nisbet was particularly interested in ideas of development and change as they were used by Western social thinkers. The idea of natural history is a crucial part of the story, for the notion that there is a natural history of civilization, or of particular social institutions, has been central to much Western thought. The same notion of natural history has been applied to the understanding of diseases, in which it has meant very much the same thing as it has in other domains of knowledge. As Nisbet observed:

> Epidemiologists and physicians continue to speak of the natural history of an epidemic or sickness (forgetting oftentimes in the process the presence of sick *people*), just as economists deal with the natural history of the business firm, sociologists with the natural history of revolutions, crowds, crime-cycles, and so on. The distinction between the actual, minutely recorded, history of a thing, and the history that we conceive as flowing from its very nature, when not deflected or otherwise interfered with,

remains a vital distinction for most of us even though we rarely today make it as explicit as did the philosophers of the eighteenth century (italics in original).[3]

This way of understanding social change and the nature of diseases in populations and individuals has been enormously valuable, for it allows one to generalize and to predict the trajectory of many phenomena. It is, however, only one version of natural history. Another is exemplified by Gilbert White, the 18th-century parson of Selborne, who wrote that he was "laying before the public his idea of *parochial history*" (italics in original). He continued, "If stationary men would pay some attention to the districts on which they reside, and would publish their thoughts respecting the objects that surround them, from such materials might be drawn the most complete county-histories."[4] The tradition of natural history of which White is an inspirational figure is grounded in intimate knowledge of particular places and the relationships among the organisms of which it is constituted. It is not universal history but local history or, as White termed it, parochial history.

In this book I should like to argue for the value of a particularistic approach to the study of diseases in populations. This is not unprecedented. Until the great scientific advances of the late 19th century, especially the bacteriological revolution, physicians were concerned primarily with the characteristics of particular patients and the characteristic diseases of particular places. In his mid-19th-century classic, *Principal Diseases of the Interior Valley of North America*, Daniel Drake wrote:

> There are diseases which occur independently of all known external influences, which affect individuals of all races, and present in all cases substantially the same symptoms and lesions of structure. . . . In reference to all these . . . it may be said, that the observations made in one country are, in the main, equally applicable to every other. The maladies are the common scourge of our race; and the knowledge of their symptoms, lesions, and treatment, the common heritage of our profession.
>
> On the other hand, there are diseases which scarcely ever occur but in certain climates, localities, or states of society. . . . Here then is the foundation of local medical history and practice; a basis which does not support the whole nosology, and yet is broad enough for a large superstructure whenever an extended region constitutes the field of enquiry.[5]

The importance of local knowledge was thought to have been made obsolete by the developments of biomedical science, particularly by the germ theory in the late 19th century and by utterances in the social sciences (stemming from the assumptions described by Nisbet) about the stages of economic and social development and modernization. In medicine—as in the social sciences—valid and valued professional knowledge has become universal knowledge.[6] I have taken a different position. It is not that I believe it is impossible or undesirable to make broad generalizations about the misfortunes that affect peoples or about the way they attempt to cope with them. Far from it. My belief is, however, that at our present stage of knowledge and in the wake of the recent collapse of many old certainties, it is likely to be more useful to understand in detail the myriad ways in which different causes of morbidity and mortality in populations are affected by social processes, rather than to strive to build grand theories.

To impose some order on such an immense topic, I have limited my discussion in the following ways: First, I shall consider only the indigenous peoples of the United States, Canada, some large Polynesian islands, and Australia. Second, I shall consider the impact of European contact and social change on the mortality and morbidity of these populations. Third, I shall be selective in the topics I cover and the examples I choose. Fourth, in most chapters I shall use the comparative method to isolate important explanatory variables.

The structure of the book moves from macrosocial international comparisons to microsocial intracultural comparisons. The points I should like to make by organizing my book in this way are several. First, diseases rarely act as independent forces but instead are shaped by the different contexts in which they occur. In this regard I describe the trajectories of population change after European contact to argue that factors other than disease were at least as significant as the introduction of new microorganisms into previously unexposed populations.

Second, preventive and curative interventions have had profound consequences for disease patterns and life expectancy, but this has not always been the case. In the instances I consider, the reasons for failure have been political and institutional, as have the reasons for success. But political institutions are themselves the products of historical forces and are not easily changed simply by an act of what is nowadays called political will.

Third, diseases differ, and different kinds of diseases have their trajectories shaped differently in different populations. In some instances it is useful to think of them as having a natural, in others a social, history.

Fourth, notions of modernization as described by Nisbet have had a great impact on the way that epidemiologists and demographers have written about changing epidemiologic regimes. It is true that many writers besides Nisbet have seriously questioned those linear theories. Nonetheless they are still important, and I argue that they are often misleading when applied to the indigenous peoples I consider in this book. The processes by which such peoples have been "modernized" are variable, as are the health consequences. In some instances it was labor that the Europeans wanted, in others land, and in still others both. Where labor and land were wanted, as in the case of Native Hawaiians, integration into the lowest social class of an emerging capitalist society occurred. When labor was not wanted, but only land, as was the case with most American Indians and Australian Aborigines, isolation on reservations and missions occurred. In these cases it is difficult to claim that integration into the class system has occurred, but rather isolation and encapsulation. And in cases in which labor but not land was wanted, as in Samoa, a typical colonial system developed, with a planter class and indigenous people continuing to live and work in their own villages. In the last two instances certain traditional behaviors persisted because they were a way of adapting to economic marginality. Such behaviors have continuing relevance to some but not all causes of morbidity and mortality.

Fifth, this book is about epistemology as much as it is about epidemiology. I am making an argument for accepting the importance of diversity and local knowledge in our understanding of diseases in populations. One reader of an early version of this book said that the emphasis on local history and the suggestion that a generalization of conclusions is impossible are a "postmodernist nihilist strategy employed by scholars who feel that their only task is to deconstruct things." That is not my position. Among people writing about health and disease, one sees the same polarization as in other aspects of our culture, between those who believe that scientific knowledge is generalizable and universally accessible and those who believe that truth is local, relative, and socially constructed. My view is that it is possible to know the world and not simply construct it but that the kind of knowledge that is useful depends on the question one wants to answer. I am concerned with diseases in populations, and I contend in this book that diseases in populations are so diverse that attempts at generalizing may often—but not always—be vacuous and go badly astray. There is still a lot of mileage to be gotten out of thinking about diseases in their local or national contexts, even understanding that some processes are universal. Generalizations may be parsimonious. They may also be impoverished.

To create a context for the detailed studies of North America and Oceania, in the remainder of this chapter I sketch briefly the contrasts between the epidemiologic and demographic consequences of European contact in Africa and the Americas and then between those in Latin and English America. The contrast between Africa and the Americas is meant to show, as many before this have done, that their different disease ecologies had a profound impact on the Europeans and on the consequences of European colonization for the native peoples. The contrast between Latin and English America is meant to illustrate that different colonial policies had different consequences as well. Clearly, disease ecology placed tighter or looser constraints on Europeans, but where the constraints were relatively loose, as in the Americas and Oceania, policy differences had quite different epidemiologic and demographic consequences.

In Chapter 2 the focus narrows to Australia, Canada, New Zealand, and the United States, all places where English-speaking liberal democracies were established. I do not deal with the history of the indigenous population decline but, rather, with the consequences for the health of the indigenous peoples of institutional and policy differences in the 20th century. My point is that different forms of federalism have had important implications both for the way that central and state governments deal with indigenous peoples and for their health. These differences have tended to be more observable in regard to infectious than to noninfectious diseases, because the health services that have been created have been better equipped to deal with infectious conditions. In general, where treaties have been signed and where the central government has assumed responsibility for relations with indigenous peoples, their general health and welfare are better than where state governments have assumed responsibility.

One of the difficulties with the analysis in Chapter 2 is that the indigenous peoples of the four nations are themselves very different. Therefore in Chapter 3 I have looked for populations that are similar in social organization and culture but that differ in regard to their historical and contemporary experiences with Europeans. I have chosen several Polynesian populations that have in common not only their biological inheritance and language but also the fact that they reside on large islands with large, stratified populations. That is, I have tried to control as best I can for genetic background, culture, and social organization while observing the effects on health of different types of European contact.

This third chapter is devoted to the history of the population since the first intensive European contact in the late 18th century. I argue that the population collapse was especially severe and prolonged on the two largest island groups, New Zealand and Hawaii, because these were places where settlers dispossessed indigenous people from their lands. Tonga and Samoa had quite different histories. But even here one finds a poorly understood anomaly, the Marquesas, where the population decline was especially severe and prolonged and where dispossession was not a significant factor. Most of Chapter 3, however, considers contemporary patterns of mortality and morbidity, which I attempt to explain by invoking a variety of political and economic factors.

Because the analyses in Chapter 2 and 3 are at a macrosocial level, it is difficult to demonstrate the details of the way that government structure and policy influence health. Thus in Chapter 4 I depart from the comparative perspective to consider in greater depth the relationships between policy and the health of Aborigines in Queensland, Australia. I have chosen this population because of all the peoples discussed in this book, the Aborigines (particularly the men) have by far the lowest life expectancy. It is therefore especially important to try to understand why. I contend first that the population decline in the 19th century was not due primarily to diseases acting independently but to the savagery with which the Aborigines were hunted and slaughtered, particularly by pastoralists and miners who were intent on occupying the land and extracting its natural resources. I then show that in the 20th century the very slow improvement in Aboriginal health has been due to the particularly dysfunctional form of federalism applied to the Aboriginal policy that has developed in Australia.

The first four chapters all are concerned with environmental factors, either natural or social, that have influenced the historical and current disease patterns of indigenous peoples. I argue that disease ecology was an important constraint historically and that when it is held roughly constant, one can see more clearly the enormous impact that different colonial and contemporary policies have had. But all these analyses ignore the very real differences among indigenous peoples and the contribution their own cultures make to shaping their disease experience.

Thus in Chapter 5 I looked for a setting in which government policy and services, as well as natural ecology, are the same but where the cultures of the people differ. All my examples are drawn from the Navajo and Hopi Indians who live as neighbors on the Colorado Plateau in the American Southwest. What I wish to demonstrate in this chapter is that people with different cultures and patterns of social organization responded to Anglo-American contact in different ways, with different consequences for their health. Moreover, I wish to show that even now culture continues to make a difference in the incidence, prevalence, and trajectory of certain conditions. It is in this context that I discuss the distinction between the concepts of the natural history of disease and the careers of patients with a disease. I argue that when attempting to explain disease trajectories, each concept has more or less utility, depending on the characteristics of the condition being considered. The comparison of the same diseases in two populations with access to the same health and welfare system helps make the point.

The discussion in Chapter 5 tends to treat the two societies as homogeneous, whereas in fact, each is rather diverse. Some of that diversity in Hopi society is dealt with there, but it is in Chapter 6 that intratribal variability is considered in greater depth. Several sources of internal differentiation among Navajos (regional, social status, and gender) and their health-related consequences are described. It is in this chapter that I address most directly the issue of "modernization" and health. I make the point that social change does not affect everyone similarly, that the differences are not random in the population, and that different measures of health and disease are useful for understanding the impact of social change among different segments and strata of the population.

I have thus organized the sequence to allow me to describe, first, the difference that disease ecology made to European colonization. Then, by focusing on English and Spanish America, I assume a relatively constant disease ecology and so am able to consider the importance of different colonial policies. Next, by discussing only English-speaking liberal democracies in temperate zones, I am able to focus on the impact of institutional arrangements on indigenous people. Then, by considering two different populations living as neighbors and influenced by the same government policies, I am able to say something about how culture influences health. Finally, by considering differences within the same population, I am able to describe how intracultural variations shape several different health consequences of European contact.

THE OLD WORLD AND THE NEW

For my purposes the Old World includes Eurasia and Africa, and the New World includes the Americas and Oceania. The expansion of Europe had an enormous impact on all non-Europeans, but epidemiologically and demographically it took a somewhat different form in each world. To the degree that European contact with non-Europeans in Asia and Africa had health-related consequences, they were the result primarily of political and economic domination. In the Americas and Oceania, by contrast, contact-induced diseases were as much a prelude to European domination as its aftermath. Here domination was facilitated, and even made possible in certain instances, by devastating pandemics that often decimated and demoralized whole populations and that on occasion spread in advance of the invading Europeans, carried by the natives who fled before them.[7]

These differences are accounted for by the fact that the diseases carried by Europeans, most notably perhaps smallpox and measles, were diseases to which they themselves had been exposed, survived, and become immune. This was true as well for large parts of Eurasia and some areas of Africa.[8] But it was not the case in the New World, where the natives had never been exposed to such diseases and where entire populations were afflicted almost simultaneously, leaving no one to carry on the vital tasks of nursing the sick and producing subsistence. Whether these people were also immunologically more vulnerable because their ancestors had never been exposed to these conditions is a matter of debate. It is plausible but not necessary to explain what happened. In so-called virgin-soil populations exposed for the first time to an acute infectious disease, everyone who is exposed gets sick. In severe diseases such as smallpox and measles, the debility may be such as to make it impossible for people to care for themselves. High deathrates, demoralization, and social collapse ensue. Often the religion of the invaders was thought (by both Europeans and natives) to be more powerful than the religious beliefs and practices of the natives, further increasing the demoralization of the natives and making conquest that much easier.

Population decline as a result of epidemics is most likely if the young are selectively affected.[9] If people of all ages are afflicted equally, as is the case in virgin-soil epidemics, then it is likely that—short of annihilation of the entire population—enough young people will remain to reproduce and begin the process of population recovery. But if the young are lost selectively, such a process cannot occur, unless of course they are obtained from elsewhere, by raiding, for example. Among the most lethal New World epidemics were smallpox and measles, acute infectious diseases that evoke lifelong immunity. Thus, after an initial epidemic of, say, smallpox in a virgin-soil population, all the survivors would be immune, but anyone born after the epidemic would be susceptible. Accordingly, if a second epidemic of the same disease struck 20 years later, everyone under 20 would very likely fall sick, and—depending on local circumstances—a high proportion would probably die. The result would be a heavy loss of young people. If the same happened in another 10 or 20 years, the results would be the same. After a while, the population would cease to reproduce itself and would decline. If more than one disease were involved, for example, both smallpox and measles, the decline would be exacerbated.

The same effect could be achieved in other ways, of course. First, mortality might disrupt marriages because of the death of one or both of the spouses. The result would be the premature termination of childbearing, as happened to the Maori after the 1918 influenza pandemic.[10] Second, children might fail to be born because one or both members of the couple are sterile, usually as the result of venereal disease. For example, Rallu calculated that among Marquesan women born between 1860 and 1886, the average number of children born was four, about half what would have been expected. He writes: "Proportions of primary infertile women, due to widespread venereal disease, were very high: 36% in generations 1860–81, whereas it is normally around 5% in populations where all the women get married, like the Marquesan."[11] Notice that women of childbearing age may be fertile but that because of the loss of members from their age cohort might still not be able to bear sufficient children to outnumber the deaths. That is, crude birthrates may be lower than crude deathrates because of infertility, a dearth of women, or both. Knowing only crude birthrates is not sufficient to distinguish between the possibilities. Third, children might be born and fail to survive because of active or passive infanticide or extraordinarily high rates of infant and child mortality due to endemic as well as epidemic diseases. None of these possibilities is mutually exclusive of the others, but estimating their relative importance in early contact and historic populations is likely to prove virtually impossible.

In addition to sharing many diseases with Europeans, non-European natives of the Old World had some unique diseases of their own to which Europeans had not been exposed. These were the so-called tropical diseases, most of which cannot flourish in temperate climates. Europeans often did poorly when exposed to such disease environments. Since the native populations of Africa and Asia were not being decimated by European diseases and since European settlers and soldiers were often weakened if not killed by the tropical diseases, the same kind of European demographic wave that engulfed the natives of the New World did not overwhelm those of the Old.[12] But this is not to say that European contact was without effect on the health of Asians and Africans. I shall draw my examples from Africa south of the Sahara because, though part of the Old World, its disease pool was not so thoroughly mixed with that of the Europeans as was the Asians' or North Africans' disease pool.

Africa

Africa south of the Sahara is a land in which a large number of chronic infectious diseases—such as typhoid, leprosy, trypanosomiasis (sleeping sickness), and malaria—are endemic and presumably have been so for centuries. Though often lethal (especially sleeping sickness), as often as not their effect is debilitating. It is generally agreed that a rough sort of equilibrium must have developed between the human and microbial populations. The human adaptations were both physiological and sociocultural, though the distinction is not always a clear one. Among physiological adaptations, by far the best known is the sickle cell trait, which enhances resistance to malaria. Among sociocultural adaptations was the tendency for trade to be carried on at the borders of territories.[13]

European colonization, beginning in the 16th century but intensifying enormously in the 19th, upset what must have been at best an unstable equilibrium. Beyond the possible introduction of new diseases,[14] European colonialism's acceleration in the 1880s caused a major disruption by forcing large groups of people to work on plantations in areas distant from their homes, usually under unhealthy and unsanitary conditions.[15] Caldwell argued that the demographic regime of premodern sub-Saharan Africa can be described as "a society where women averaged 5.5–7 live births yielding a birth rate of 42–50 per thousand, and where the expectation of life at birth was 20–30 years yielding a death rate of 38–50 per thousand and an infant mortality rate of 250–375 per thousand live births."[16] Until the 1880s, he continues, the "clearest assault on the demographic balance" was the slave trade.[17] Beginning in the 1880s when the race for colonies intensified, long-distance trade and troop movements became increasingly frequent. Moreover, the shift from subsistence farming to the monocropping of cash crops for sale in the world market led to landlessness, urban migration, and deteriorating nutritional status. Though adequate registration data are not available, the far from unanimous consensus is that the colonial period, beginning in the late 19th century, saw a deterioration of the health situation in southern Africa.

One of the most interesting and significant consequences of this period was the creation in Central Africa of a region of high infertility. For my purposes in this book, it is significant because it shows that the same diseases may have quite different consequences depending on the culture of the people afflicted. In this instance, as the Caldwells found, a striking feature of the pattern of sterility is its ethnic specificity. "The evidence is far from complete," they write, "but almost all that does exist points in the same direction; where sterility exists, the society does not attempt so strongly to prevent premarital sexual relations. Such societies also seem to be marked by higher marital instability, but, of course, the break-up of marriages may be the result of sterility as well as the cause of it."[18] They continue:

> The picture is then one of new diseases (or new strains of disease) entering an area previously largely isolated. The diseases were venereal in the sense that they were transmitted by sexual relations and they had their most devastating effect where there was a certain freedom in sexual relations. They entered the country just at a time when European colonization was causing substantial movements of population, particularly of men without women.[19]

They concluded that in a population where the average age at first marriage is 16, primary sterility occurred as a result of gonorrheal infections contracted at age 10 or 12.[20] Thus the impact of colonial rule in Africa was observed in patterns of both mortality and fertility, and they differed among populations depending on location, culture, and type of contact.

Paradoxically, during the postcolonial era, attempts at economic development have often had the untoward effect of worsening the health situation in ways not unlike those of the colonial era. For example, damming rivers in Ghana has expanded the zone of river blindness (onchocerciasis). Road construction in Liberia; migrant labor from Upper Volta, Mali, and Niger to southern Ghana; and settlement relocation from high plateaus to lowland agricultural areas in northern Nigeria all have been implicated in the dissemination of sleeping sickness.[21] The construction of irrigation systems has resulted in the spread of schistosomiasis and malaria. Diamond and gold mining in South Africa have caused the spread of venereal disease and tuberculosis, as well as the disruption of families.[22] AIDS is only the latest, and surely not the last, in a long list of epidemiologic disasters that have resulted from the disruption of African life since the intrusion of Europeans.

Even though disease control programs have helped improve health in some regions and one major killer—smallpox—has been eradicated, life expectancy has increased only modestly since World War II, and infant and child mortality remain high. Indeed, close to half of all deaths occur among children under the age of 5 years, the vast majority from infectious and parasitic diseases and diseases of the respiratory system, followed by diseases of the digestive system.[23] A number of reasons have been proposed, including impoverishment, inflation, international indebtedness, natural disasters, warfare, and less aid from abroad,[24] all of which are causes of infant and child malnutrition.

In summary, the health of Africans worsened and then has improved only slowly since the time of intense colonization by Europeans in the 19th century. Much is accounted for by the nature of Africa's disease ecology, but it seems safe to say that the spread of epidemics and the presumed deterioration of life expectancy followed on the heels of the Europeans' assertion of social and political control.

The Americas

This situation was reversed in the New World, where social, political, and economic domination by Europeans followed on the heels of epidemics. Here the epidemiologic and demographic consequences of European contact were even more catastrophic for the indigenous populations than they were for the indigenous Africans.[25]

The New World encountered by Spanish, Portuguese, English, French, and other explorers and colonists was highly diverse, both ecologically and culturally. It encompassed arctic, temperate, and tropical climates; small bands of hunter-gatherers and large complex empires based on irrigation and agriculture; low-lying river basins and high mountain ranges. I shall consider some of the consequences of that diversity in subsequent chapters. Here I shall point to the similarities. For no matter where they lived, no matter how sophisticated their cultures, no matter how complex their social organization and technology, the overwhelming fact is that demographic decline, if not complete collapse, was the fate of virtually all indigenous groups in the Americas.

Acute infectious diseases introduced by Europeans, most notably smallpox, measles, and perhaps influenza, played an important role in this decline.[26] Indigenous Americans had evidently not been exposed to these diseases previously, perhaps because the animal hosts in which they first evolved and from which they spread to humans were not present in the Western Hemisphere[27] or perhaps because even large aboriginal populations were too isolated to sustain such diseases.[28] These diseases were followed by others, some transmitted directly by the Europeans (such as typhus and diphtheria), others by African slaves (such as malaria, yellow fever, and hookworm).

Other factors were important as well, however.[29] For example, some authorities believe that tuberculosis had existed in the precontact indigenous population but became a major killer only when the hardships and stress of European contact and domination made themselves felt.[30] Other causes of depopulation were famine induced by the destruction and/or confiscation of crops by the invaders, forced labor in mines and on plantations, warfare, the absence of marriage partners (both a cause and a consequence of depopulation), and epidemic-induced panic, social disorganization, and demoralization. The question about which there has been much debate is the degree to which diseases acted independently of these other factors. I shall leave that aside for now and return to it in Chapters 3 and 4. There I shall argue that disease was not a deus ex machina but that the kind of contact that occurred was of great significance. Essentially, when displacement from land—often accompanied by warfare—occurred, the results were especially catastrophic.

Though the fact of demographic decline is widely acknowledged, its magnitude and timing have been a fruitful source of disagreement and debate.[31] There are a variety of ways of estimating the aboriginal population.[32] They result in very different figures for the 1490s, the time of the first significant European contact, from a low of 8.4 million to a high of 112 million.[33] The higher the initial figure the greater the magnitude of subsequent loss to the nadir. Indeed, some authorities believe that the loss of population across the entire Western Hemisphere was over 90 percent. Others argue that the depopulation was much smaller, conceivably even less than 50 percent.

The writers who believe the numbers at contact were very high contend that disease was the major cause of decline and that much of the collapse occurred in the 16th century before face-to-face contact between most Indians and Europeans but as a result of the diffusion of epidemics. Low counters have tended to minimize the impact of disease. The debate is significant because the high counters argue that the social organization before the collapse was very different from what it was afterward, and thus ethnographic and historical reconstructions of precontact populations must necessarily be wrong.

The available evidence suggests that disease was in fact important, as I have argued, but that inferences about the size of the population at contact are extremely uncertain. The high counts are based on backward projections from population nadirs and assume ratios of population at contact that were at least 20 times greater than the nadir populations. Such inferences assume a natural history of epidemics that was everywhere the same. In the case of the Navajo and Hopi Indians (described in Chapter 5) and the Polynesians (described in Chapter 3), this does not seem to have been so. Nor does it seem to have been true on the Northern Plains,[34] among the Iroquois of central New York State, or among the Pueblos along the Rio Grande.[35] Indeed, in regard to the Indians north of the great civilizations of Mexico, the decline to nadir seems to have ranged from a high of 95 percent among the California Indians to a low of 53 and 56 percent in the Arctic and sub-Arctic, respectively.[36]

The point of this comparison between Africa and the Americas is that disease ecology had profound consequences for both the invading Europeans and the indigenous peoples. It shaped the way the Europeans were able to colonize Africa and the New World, and it influenced the epidemiologic and demographic responses of the indigenous peoples they encountered. At the same time, the policies pursued by Europeans colonizers and settlers also had far-reaching epidemiologic and demographic consequences.

SPANISH AND ENGLISH AMERICA

Numerous observers have commented on the differences between the Spanish and English colonization of the New World. According to McAlister,[37] one formulation has it that "whereas the English came to America to settle and till the soil, the Spaniards came only to plunder." But, he continues, there was far more to Spanish policy than that, for although plunder was indeed intended and occurred, the concern was also to create a "Christian republic where men lived in polity and justice *according to their rank and station* and made the land bear fruit" (italics added). I have emphasized "rank and station" because race—Indianness—became in Spanish America a measure of both and the lowest of each. For the Spanish the availability of Indian labor—first for work in the mines and ultimately for work on the haciendas—was crucial.

Patterns of land tenure and social stratification that developed in the colonial period persisted in the 19th century even as the demand for Latin American exports resulted in economic growth.

> The colonial period was thus responsible for establishing the pattern of large land-holdings and an exploited peasant or slave underclass throughout much of Latin America. The availability and reliability of commercial opportunities clearly had much to do with the location and characteristics of the productive systems that emerged. During this period, economic and demographic changes had direct consequences for the use of land, labor, and capital in the region. Underlying these changes, however, was a striking uniformity in the unequal distribution of land and the dependent position of labor, whether in areas dominated by domestic production or in those dominated by export production. In the nineteenth century, commercial expansion changed the nature of many agricultural enterprises in the region. Export markets came to dominate production, foreign money flowed into the sector, and export profits stimulated national economies. If anything, however, these changes further cemented the nature of land-holding and rural power relations that had developed in the colonial period.[38]

Indeed, the concentration of landholding increased right into the present century. The economic collapse of the 1930s worked a significant change, however, because the national governments in Latin America began to assume a more central role in the organization of the economy. It was then that social welfare programs began to be introduced and government-led drives for industrial development first emerged.[39] The development ideology that gave intellectual legitimacy to the governments' plans included "import substitution," a major role for government planning and direction, and a central place for agricultural modernization "to support and finance industrial development."[40]

The modernization of agriculture required investment in infrastructure—tractors, new seeds, fertilizers, and so on—and the "efficient" use of land, which was generally understood to mean the consolidation of already large haciendas, plantations, and ranches; the dispossession of many small landholders; the exacerbation of rural insecurity and landlessness for the majority of peasants; and rapid urbanization.

It began to be clear in the 1960s that these policies were having some untoward consequences in regard to rural unrest, most impressively in the success of the Cuban revolution in 1959. As a result of that revolution, "95 percent of landholdings over 67 hectares in size were expropriated from private owners . . . and were turned into state farms and cooperatives."[41] Several other countries also engaged in land redistribution as a result of revolution, but most of the redistribution was carried out from above by national governments. No doubt the fear of revolution and the encouragement of the Kennedy administration played an important role, but it was also thought that only land redistribution would counteract the inefficiencies of the existing pattern and result in true capitalist farming.

Land reform was clearly unpopular among the vested interests, however, and the result was that it was halted, often by military takeovers of national governments, as in Chile in 1973. Thus in the 1970s, a "nondistributional approach to rural poverty" was attempted, with the encouragement of the World Bank under its then president, Robert McNamara.

> Generally, programs were designed with three components: (1) direct inputs to improve production (usually given the largest portion of program funds); (2) infrastructure to encourage and support increased production; and (3) social infrastructure such as health and educational facilities and peasant organizations (usually given the smallest portion of program funds). The approach largely avoided the issue of redistribution of land, indicating that goods and services could be provided that would enable the peasant to produce more at a greater profit; these could be applied without altering the structure of landholding and would still have a significant impact on the standard of living in rural areas.[42]

This brief sketch has ignored substantial differences within Latin America. For example, not all of Mexico and South and Central America was occupied by extensive indigenous agricultural societies, and where mobile hunting–gathering tribes were found, domination was much more difficult—even impossible—to impose. In vast areas of tropical forest in northern Brazil, no European settlements were established. In some tropical areas, slaves from Africa were introduced, primarily into the Caribbean islands and along the northeast and northern Pacific coasts of South America.[43] Grassland areas in what became Argentina, Uruguay, and southern Brazil had no extensive indigenous agriculture and hence did not attract early Spanish settlement. As Oveido, a Spanish chronicler, commented, "The Indies are worth nothing without the Indians." Indeed, it was these areas that attracted the greatest amount of European immigration during the late 19th century.[44]

The policy in English America was different: "The British, unlike their rivals, the French and the Spaniards, never developed an overall eighteenth-century colonial policy that gave the Indian a place and a future in the structure of the empire."[45] Indians were widely viewed as savages to be dominated and eliminated, and the epidemics that decimated the Indians were widely considered to be evidence of God's favor. As savages, Indians were supposed inevitably to give way to a higher civilization.[46] It was only in the late 19th century—not coincidentally at the same time that Anglo-Americans began to worry about the preservation of their natural environment and to create national parks—that concern about the survival of American Indians began to be expressed and for that expression to find its way very slowly into policy. But by then the Indians in the eastern half of the country had been largely exterminated, and their remnants placed on small, fragmented reservations overseen by state governments. In the West, however, sizable Indian populations still survived, and their treaties were made with the federal government. They were placed on reservations that as the 20th century wore on, and particularly after the 1930s, were increasingly well protected legally and well served medically, though their natural resources were generally extracted by, and in the interests of, others.

What, then, were the consequences for the Indians' health of these different colonial policies? Of course, all of Latin America is far more diverse than the United States and Canada; demographic responses to contact differed widely from one place to another within Latin America;[47] and data on the Indians' health status are harder to find there than in North America. In general, however, the effect of the contrasting policies has been that the health of North American Indians has improved far more rapidly than has that of Indians in Latin America. In Latin America throughout the 19th century, and in some countries into the present century as well, mortality from both endemic and epidemic diseases was very high. As late as the 1920s and 1930s, for example, studies in Guatemala and the Yucatán Peninsula found that infant mortality had reached extraordinary levels, that malnutrition was common, that enteric diseases were caused by a bewildering assortment of microorganisms, and that malaria was epidemic.[48] This was an area of dense Indian settlement, much of it in free villages that had escaped land enclosures.[49] Population growth and presumably the local system of social stratification had resulted in the division of property into dwarf holdings and necessitated labor migration—often to lowland coffee plantations—to supplement local subsistence agriculture. This situation is not unique to highland Guatemala. Oscar Lewis pointed out that Mexican history is often conceived of as a conflict between haciendas and free villages, that even in free villages there was a high proportion of landless peasants, and that even those with land often had holdings so small that they needed to find other sources of income as well.[50] It is this constellation of landlessness, labor migration, and rural poverty that is associated with high mortality throughout much of Latin America. In general, rural mortality is higher than urban mortality in all countries for which data have been published,[51] the reverse of the 19th-century North American and North European patterns, and a number of studies suggest that involvement in agricultural wage labor is associated with higher rates of morbidity and mortality than is the relatively greater dependence on subsistence farming.[52]

Moreover, data from Bolivia, Ecuador, and Guatemala in the 1970s show that the probability of death at various ages is greater for Indians than non-Indians, even when urban–rural residence and educational attainment of the mother (in the case of infant and child mortality) are statistically controlled.[53] Infant and child mortality in a rural Zapotec Indian community in Mexico was substantially higher, though falling, in the period between 1945 and 1970 than was infant and child mortality in all of Mexico and was similar to rates reported from highland Maya Indian communities.[54] Moreover, adult heights showed no increase over those of the previous century, indicating no improvement in nutritional status.[55] And studies of body composition and growth of Cakchiquel Indian children in Guatemala demonstrate no improvement in nutritional status over a period of two decades and suggest reduced nutritional reserves when compared with those of non-Indian children.[56] These data reveal a continuing pattern of death in infancy and childhood due to endemic infectious diseases and malnutrition. On the other hand, there is some evidence that Indian mortality is dropping in some areas and is converging with non-Indian mortality rates.[57]

The situation evolved somewhat differently in the United States. Compared with all U.S. races, Indians have twice the unemployment rate, half the per capita income, and less than half the proportion of college graduates. On the other hand, life expectancy and causes of death have been changing dramatically. I shall discuss this issue in more detail in the next chapter. Suffice it to say here that for both sexes the rate of improvement in life expectancy since the 1940s has been more than twice as rapid for Indians as for whites but that Indian life expectancy still lags by about 3 years for each sex.[58] At ages below 44, Indians die at greater rates than does the rest of the population. Between 45 and 64, the rates are the same. At 65 and above, Indians die at lower rates. This pattern is the result of differences in the relative importance of various causes of death among Indians and non-Indians. Among Indians over the past 30 to 40 years, infectious diseases have declined in significance; cancer and cardiovascular diseases are not as significant as they are among non-Indians; and violence and substance abuse have remained higher among Indians and account for most of the difference in life expectancy at birth.[59]

The colonial policies of Spain and England have had a great impact both on the subsequent economic development of Latin America and the United States and on policies regarding the treatment of Indians. The Spanish policy was to incorporate Indians as the lowest social stratum of the polity. In combination with the generally low level of economic development characteristic of most Latin American countries, the result has been a persistent pattern of high infant mortality and deaths from endemic infectious diseases. In the United States, on the other hand, the great wealth of the country, the special status that Indians ultimately achieved, and the provision of services on reservations have not resulted in dramatically improved economic conditions but have resulted in the control of infectious diseases and malnutrition and the emergence of noninfectious diseases and violence as the most important causes of reduced life expectancy.

The decline of mortality from epidemic diseases in Latin America and from epidemic and endemic infectious diseases in North America has enabled the growth of the Indian population. I have already said that there is much disagreement surrounding estimates of the number of Indians living in the Americas at the time of first contact. It is equally difficult to arrive at a figure for the present Indian population, since "Indian" is as much a social as a biological designation.[60] Keeping in mind the difficulties of estimation and enumeration, it is still useful to suggest what the magnitude of change may have been from the 1490s to the present. Somewhat conservative estimates for the early period are as follows: North America, 4.4 million; Central America, 21.4 million; and South America, 20 million.[61] Estimates for the 1960s and 1970s are North America, 1.5 million to 2.0 million;[62] Central America, 5.0 million; and South America, 10 million.[63]

It is generally agreed that the low point of the Latin American Indian population occurred in the 17th and 18th centuries.[64] The population then began to increase as a result of the decline of epidemics, especially in the 19th century. Improvements in medical care and public health seem not to have played much of a role until well into the 20th century.[65] The low point of the North American Indian population occurred around the turn of the present century.[66] By the late 20th century there had been substantial recovery all across the Western Hemisphere, though some tribes had become extinct and the cultures of the surviving tribes had been irrevocably changed. Thus the population history of Latin America is to a very large degree the history of the indigenous population. In the population history of English America, the indigenous people are only a small part of the story, both because the numbers and complexity of the indigenous societies in Latin America were orders of magnitude greater than in English America and because the colonial policies of the invading nations differed immensely.

CONCLUSION

In this chapter I argued that disease ecology had very different consequences for the colonial experience in Africa and the Americas and that only by holding roughly constant the disease ecology does the impact of differing colonial policies become readily observable. Indeed, throughout the Western Hemisphere and Oceania—where the preexisting disease regimes did not place as severe constraints on Europeans as they did in sub-Saharan Africa—the health consequences of differing colonial policies are particularly visible. It is to some of those patterns that I turn in the following chapters.

NOTES

1. R. Nisbet, *Social Change and History: Aspects of the Western Theory of Development* (Oxford: Oxford University Press, 1969), p. 140.

2. Ibid., p. 140.

3. Ibid., pp. 157–58.

4. G. White, *The Natural History of Selborne* (1789) (New York: Dutton, 1971), p. 1. See also D. Worster, *Nature's Economy: A History of Ecological Ideas* (Cambridge: Cambridge University Press, 1985).

5. D. Drake, *A Systematic Treatise, Historical, Etiological, and Practical, on the Principal Diseases of the Interior Valley of North America* (Cincinnati: Winthrop B. Smith, 1850), pp. 1–2.

6. See S. J. Kunitz, "Explanations and ideologies of mortality patterns," *Population and Development Review* 13 (1987): 379–408; S. J. Kunitz, "Hookworm and pellagra: Exemplary diseases in the New South," *Journal of Health and Social Behavior* 29 (1988): 139–48.

7. W. W. Borah, "America as a model: The demographic impact of European expansion upon the non-European world," Actas y Memorias, Thirty-fifth Congreso Internacional de Americanistas, Mexico City, 1962. 1964. See also A. F. Ramenofsky, *Vectors of Death* (Albuquerque: University of New Mexico Press, 1987).

8. When Europe first began trading with Japan in the 1860s, no epidemics ensued, because the Japanese, unlike the population of the New World, had been exposed to the same pool of infectious diseases as had the Europeans themselves, and for just as long. See A. B. Janetta, *Epidemics and Mortality in Early Modern Japan* (Princeton, NJ: Princeton University Press, 1987).

9. N. McArthur, *Island Populations of the Pacific* (Canberra: Australian National University Press, 1968).

10. D. I. Pool, *Te Iwi Maori: A New Zealand Population Past, Present and Projected* (Auckland: University of Auckland Press, 1991), p. 118.

11. J. L. Rallu, "Population of the French overseas territories in the Pacific, past, present and projected," *Journal of Pacific History* 26 (1991): 170.

12. G. W. Hartwig and K. D. Patterson, eds., *Disease in African History: An Introductory Survey and Case Studies* (Durham, NC: Duke University Press, 1978).

13. M. J. Azevadeo, "Epidemic disease among the Sara of southern Chad, 1890–1940," in Hartwig and Patterson, eds., *Disease in African History,* pp. 118–52.

14. J. R. Dias, "Famine and disease in the history of Angola c. 1830–1930," *Journal of African History* 22 (1981): 349–78.

15. M. W. DeLancey, "Health and disease on the plantation of Cameroon, 1884–1939," in Hartwig and Patterson, eds., *Disease in African History,* pp. 153–79.

16. J. C. Caldwell, "The social repercussions of colonial rule: Demographic aspects," in A. Adu Boahen, ed., *General History of Africa* (published for UNESCO) (London: Heinemann, 1981), p. 463.

17. Ibid., p. 465.

18. J. C. Caldwell and P. Caldwell, "The demographic evidence for the incidence and cause of abnormally low fertility in tropical Africa," *World Health Statistics Quarterly* 36 (1983): 8.

19. Ibid., p. 10.

20. Primary sterility is sterility that occurs sufficiently early that a woman bears no children at all, in contrast with secondary sterility, which occurs later in life after a woman has had several births. Ibid., p. 12.

21. C. C. Hughes and J. M. Hunter, "Disease and 'development' in Africa," *Social Science and Medicine* 3 (1970): 443–93.

22. S. Kark, "The social pathology of syphilis in Africans," *South African Medical Journal* 23 (1949): 77–84; S. Kark and J. Cassel, "The Pholela health centre: A progress report," *South African Medical Journal* 26 (1952): 101–4, 131–36.

23. United Nations, *Levels and Trends of Mortality Since 1950,* Report ST/ESA/SER, A/74 (New York: Department of International Economic and Social Affairs, 1982), pp. 95–96; United Nations, *Mortality and Health Policy,* Report ST/ESA/SER/, A/91 (New York: Department of International Economic and Social Affairs, 1984).

24. A. Adediji, "Foreign debt and prospects for growth in Africa during the 1980s," *Journal of Modern African Studies* 23 (1985): 53–74.

25. Borah, "America as a Model."

26. H. Dobyns, "An outline of Andean epidemic history to 1720," *Bulletin of the History of Medicine* 37 (1963): 493–515; A. Crosby, *The Columbian Exchange: Biological and Cultural Consequences of 1492* (Westport, CT: Greenwood Press, 1972); A. Crosby, *Ecological Imperialism: The Biological Expansion of Europe, 900–1900* (Cambridge: Cambridge University Press, 1986); M. Newman, "Aboriginal new world epidemiology and medical care, and the impact of old world disease imports," *American Journal of Physical Anthropology* 45 (1976): 667–72; D. R. Snow and K. M. Lanphear, "European contact and Indian depopulation in the Northeast: The timing of the first epidemics," *Ethnohistory* 35 (1988): 15–33.

27. W. H. McNeill, *Plagues and Peoples* (Harmondsworth: Penguin Books, 1976).

28. Ramenofsky, *Vectors of Death*, p. 169.

29. See, for example, E. R. Wolf, *Europe and the People Without History* (Berkeley and Los Angeles: University of California Press, 1990), pp. 133–35.

30. J. Buikstra, ed., *Prehistoric Tuberculosis in the Americas* (Evanston, IL: Northwestern University Archaeological Program, 1981).

31. See, for instance, D. Henige, "Standards of proof and discursive strategies in the debate over Native American population at contact," In M. P. Nieto eds., *The Peopling of the Americas,* vol. 1, Proceedings of the IUSSP Conference at Veracruz, Mexico, May 17–23, 1992 (Liege, Belgium: International Union for the Scientific Study of Population, 1992), pp. 17–46.

32. R. Thornton, *American Indian Holocaust and Survival: A Population History Since 1492* (Norman: University of Oklahoma Press, 1987), pp. 21–22.

33. W. M. Deneven, ed., *The Native Population of the Americas in 1492* (Madison: University of Wisconsin Press, 1976), p. 3.

34. J. F. Decker, "Depopulation of the Northern Plains natives," *Social Science and Medicine* 33 (1991): 381–93.

35. Ramenofsky, *Vectors of Death,* pp. 165–66; A. M. Palkovich, "Historic population of the Eastern Pueblos: 1540–1910," *Journal of Anthropological Research* 41 (1985): 401–26. See also D. F. Stannard, "The consequences of contact: Toward an interdisciplinary theory of native responses to biological and cultural invasion," in D. H. Thomas, ed., *Columbian Consequences, vol. 3: The Spanish Borderlands in Pan-American Perspective* (Washington, DC: Smithsonian Institution Press, 1991), pp. 519–54.

36. D. H. Ubelaker, "North American Indian population size, A.D. 1500 to 1985," *American Journal of Physical Anthropology* 77 (1988): 289–94.

37. L. N. McAlister, *Spain and Portugal in the New World, 1492–1700* (Minneapolis: University of Minnesota Press, 1984), p. 108.

38. M. S. Grindle, *State and Countryside: Development Policy and Agrarian Politics in Latin America* (Baltimore: Johns Hopkins University Press, 1986), p. 34.

39. Ibid., p. 45.

40. Ibid., p. 48.

41. Ibid., p. 138.

42. Ibid., pp. 161–62.

43. N. Sanchez-Albornoz, *The Population of Latin America: A History* (Berkeley and Los Angeles: University of California Press, 1974), p. 138.

44. J. C. Crossley, "The River Plate countries," in H. Blakemore and C. T. Smith, eds., *Latin America: Geographic Perspectives* (London: Methuen, 1971), p. 401.

45. W. R. Jacobs, "British-colonial attitudes and policies toward the Indian in the American colonies," in H. Peckham and C. Gibson, eds., *Attitudes of Colonial Powers Toward the American Indian* (Salt Lake City: University of Utah Press, 1969), p. 100. See also L. Hanke, *Aristotle and the American Indians* (Bloomington: Indiana University Press, 1959), p. 99.

46. R. H. Pearce, *Savagism and Civilization* (Baltimore: Johns Hopkins University Press, 1965).

47. L. Newson, "Indian population patterns in colonial Spanish America," *Latin American Research Review* 20 (1985): 41–75.

48. G. C. Shattuck, *The Peninsula of Yucatan: Medical, Biological, Meteorological and Sociological Studies* (Washington, DC: Carnegie Institution of Washington, 1933); G. C. Shattuck, *A Medical Survey of the Republic of Guatemala* (Washington, DC: Carnegie Institution of Washington, 1938).

49. D. J. Fox, "Central America, including Panama," in Blakemore and Smith, eds., *Latin America*, p. 121.

50. O. Lewis, *Life in a Mexican Village: Tepotzian Restudied* (Urbana: University of Illinois Press, 1951), pp. 126–27. See also L. Crandon-Malamud, *From the Fat of Our Souls: Social Change, Political Process and Medical Pluralism in Bolivia* (Berkeley and Los Angeles: University of California Press, 1991).

51. United Nations, *Levels and Trends of Mortality Since 1950*.

52. A. C. Laurell, J. B. Gil, T. Machetto, J. Polomo, C. P. Ruffo, M. R. Chavez, M. Urbina, and N. Velazquez, "Disease and rural development: A sociological analysis of morbidity in two Mexican villages," *International Journal of Health Services* 7 (1977): 401–23; C. G. Victoria and N. Blank, "Epidemiology of infant mortality in Rio Grande do Sul, Brazil," *Journal of Tropical Medicine and Hygiene* 83 (1980): 177–86.

53. United Nations, *Levels and Trends of Mortality Since 1950*, p. 169.

54. N. S. Scrimshaw, M. A. Guzman, and J. E. Gordon, "Nutrition and infection field study in Guatemalan villages, 1959–1964: I. Study plan and experimental design," *Archives of Environmental Health* 14 (1967): 657–62; J. D. Early, "The structure and change of mortality in a Maya community," *Milbank Memorial Fund Quarterly* 48 (1970): 179–201.

55. R. M. Malina and J. H. Himes, "Patterns of childhood mortality and growth status in a rural Zapotec community," *Annals of Human Biology* 5 (1978): 517–31.

56. B. Bogin and R. B. MacVean, "Growth status of non-agrarian, semi-urban living Indians in Guatemala," *Human Biology* 56 (1984): 527–38.

57. J. D. Early, *The Demographic Structure and Evolution of a Peasant System: The Guatemalan Population* (Boca Raton: University Presses of Florida, 1982), p. 53.

58. Indian Health Service, *Trends in Indian Health—1989: Tables* (Rockville, MD: Division of Program Statistics, Office of Planing, Evaluation and Legislation, Public Health Service, Department of Health and Human Services, 1989), p. 41.

59. A broadly similar pattern is observed among Canadian Indians. See T. K. Young, *Health Care and Cultural Change: The Indian Experience in the Central Subarctic* (Toronto: University of Toronto Press, 1988), pp. 48–52.

60. Thornton, *American Indian Holocaust*, pp. 186–88.

61. Denevan, *The Native Population*, p. 291.

62. Thornton, *American Indian Holocaust*, pp. 223, 244.

63. F. M. Salzano, "Survey of the unacculturated Indians of Central and South America," in PAHO, *Biomedical Challenges Presented by the American Indian* (Washington, DC: Pan American Health Organization, 1968), pp. 60–61. More recent estimates for Latin America are substantially higher: Mesoamerica, 18.75 million; the Andes region, 17.32 million; Amazonia, 2.15 million; the Southern Cone, 1.35 million; and the Caribbean, 0.16 million. These estimates are from S. Nahmad, "Survival of Amerindians," data presented at the IUSSP conference, The Peopling of the Americas, May 17–23, 1992, Veracruz, Mexico.

64. L. Newson, *The Cost of Conquest: Indian Decline in Honduras Under Spanish Rule* (Boulder, CO: Westview Press, 1986), p. 330; W. G. Lovell, *Conquest and Survival in Colonial Guatemala: A Historical Geography of the Cuchumatan Highlands 1500–1821* (Kingston and Montreal: McGill–Queen's University Press, 1985), p. 146.

65. S. J. Kunitz, "Mortality Since Malthus," in D. Coleman and R. Schofield, eds., *The State of Population Theory* (Oxford: Blackwell, 1986), pp. 279–302.

66. Thornton, *American Indian Holocaust*, p. 159.

2

Death in the Fourth World

Every Englishman is born with a certain miraculous power
that makes him master of the world. When he wants a thing,
he never tells himself that he wants it. He waits patiently
until there comes into his mind, no one knows how, a
burning conviction that it is his moral and religious duty to
conquer those who possess the thing he wants. Then he
becomes irresistible. Like the aristocrat, he does what pleases
him and grabs what he covets: like the shopkeeper, he
pursues his purpose with the industry and steadfastness that
comes from strong religious conviction and deep sense of
moral responsibility. He is never at a loss for an effective
moral attitude. As the great champion of freedom and
national independence, he conquers and annexes half the
world, and calls it Colonization. When he wants a new
market for his adulterated Manchester goods, he sends a
missionary to teach the natives the Gospel of Peace. The
natives kill the missionary: he flies to arms in defence of
Christianity; fights for it; conquers for it; and takes the
market as a reward from heaven.

G. B. SHAW, *MAN OF DESTINY*

The peoples who are the subject of this chapter—the indigenous peoples of
Australia, Canada, New Zealand, and the United States—have much in common, and it is these commonalities that the comparisons seek to "control." They
all are members of what has been called the Fourth World: indigenous peoples
submerged by an invading society.[1] They all were colonized by the British. All
are citizens of liberal Western democracies. The countries they inhabit all contain
substantial temperate zones that attracted large numbers of Europeans. The ecological transformations caused by the introduction of Old World fauna and flora
are said to have been similar. The native peoples were much reduced by the
introduction of new diseases as well as by warfare and vigilantism. And finally,
despite horrific losses, they all have recovered substantially over the past several
generations.[3]

But if these similarities are significant, so too are the differences. First, the
indigenous people differed among and within what became the four nation-states.
Australian Aborigines, though covering a vast and ecologically diverse continent

and having hundreds of different languages, were essentially all band-level hunt-ing and gathering people. The Maoris of New Zealand lived in stratified, warlike tribes and engaged in agriculture as well as hunting and fishing. The Indians of English North America were highly diverse and included both sedentary agri-culturalists living in stratified societies and egalitarian hunting–gathering bands. After the Europeans introduced livestock, some of the Indians became pastoral-ists, and others became mounted warriors and hunters.

Second, the founding colonists themselves represented what Louis Hartz[4] calls the different "fragments" of English society: middle-class religious dissenters in what became the United States, Anglican loyalists in Canada, convicts in Austra-lia, and a combination of Australians and middle-class English in New Zealand.[5]

Third, the economic and political development of the colonies differed. The United States gained independence and became a leading capitalist industrial world power. The other three remained part of the British Commonwealth and developed what has been called "dominion capitalism," a dependence on the extraction of raw materials and their very early processing for sale, first in England and more recently in the world markets.[6]

Fourth, each of the Commonwealth countries developed public schemes for ensuring financial accessability to medical care, whether national health insur-ance (Australia and Canada) or direct provision (New Zealand), whereas the United States did not. And finally and more speculatively, the indigenous peo-ples themselves may differ physiologically in important ways. Clearly, with more variables than cases, causal inferences can only be suggestive, but I shall argue that the major determinant of differences in contemporary health are the different ways in which governments have dealt with indigenous peoples.

THE DECLINE OF MORTALITY DUE TO INFECTIOUS DISEASES

Though the data are incomplete, the trajectory of mortality decline seems to have been roughly comparable in all these Fourth World populations, but there have been some revealing differences. Table 2-1 displays the available data on life expectancy at birth for as far back in the 20th century as I could find information. Table 2-2 shows more detailed information on life expectancy at birth in the 1980s, and Table 2-3 lists infant mortality rates for the past several decades.[7] (For a discussion of data sources and quality, see Appendix 2-1.)

Several points are noteworthy. First, in no case does the life expectancy of indigenous peoples match that of nonindigenous peoples, though impressive gains have been made. This is crucial. I will be emphasizing differences in the experiences of indigenous peoples, but this very important similarity must not be forgotten.

Second, though the data are sparse, the evidence suggests that male and female life expectancy among Maoris and American Indians began to diverge in the 1940s. This is the time when antibiotics and blood replacement began to reduce maternal mortality significantly, and so it is likely that these contributed substantially to the more rapid reduction in female deaths.

Table 2–1 Life expectancy at birth, various indigenous peoples, 1920s to 1980s

Year	Maoris[a] Male	Female	U.S. Indians[b] Male	Female	Canadian Indians[c] Male	Female	Aborigines[d] Male	Female
1920s	47	45	N.A.	N.A.	N.A.	N.A.	N.A.	N.A.
1930s	46	46	N.A.	N.A.	N.A.	N.A.	N.A.	N.A.
1940s	48	54	51.3	51.9	N.A.	N.A.	N.A.	N.A.
1950s	57	58	58.1	62.2	N.A.	N.A.	N.A.	N.A.
1960s	61	65	60	65.7	59.6	63.5	50 (Northern Territory)	
1970s	63	67	60.7	71.2	57.8	60.3 (Alberta)	N.A.	N.A.
1980s	65	68	67.1	75.1	64	72.8	54	61.6

[a]E. W. Pomare, *Maori Standards of Health: A Study of the 20 Year Period 1955–1975* (Auckland: Medical Research Council of New Zealand, Special Report Series no. 7, 1980); E. W. Pomare and G. de Boer, *Hauora: Maori Standards of Health, A Study of the Years 1970–1984* (Auckland: Medical Research Council of New Zealand, Special Report Series no. 78, 1988); I. Pool, "Mortality trends and differentials," in Population of New Zealand (Banjkok: Economic and Social Commission for Asia and the Pacific, 1985).

[b]Indian Health Service, *Trends in Indian Health—1989. Tables* (Rockville, MD: Division of Program Statistics, Office of Planning, Evaluation and Legislation, Public Health Service, Department of Health and Human Services, 1989).

[c]W. J. Millar, "Mortality patterns in a Canadian Indian Population," Canadian Studies in Population 9 (1982):17–31; Ministry of National Health and Welfare, *Health Indicators Derived from Vital Statistics for Status Indian and Canadian Populations, 1978–1986* (Ottawa: Ministry of National Health and Welfare, September 1988); Medical Services, Department of National Health and Welfare, "Life tables, registered Canadian Indians, 1960–64" (Ottawa: Department of National Health and Welfare, n.d.). The registered Indian population of Alberta is about 12 to 13 percent of all registered Indians.

[d]N. J. Thomson, "Inequalities in aboriginal health" (M.P.H. thesis, University of Sydney, 1989), p. 39; A. Gray, "Discovering determinants of Australian aboriginal population health," working paper (Canberra: National Centre for Epidemiology and Population Health, Australian National University, 1989), p. 11.

Third, Aboriginal life expectancy does not differ markedly across the entire continent; it is lower than the life expectancy of any other indigenous population; and Aboriginal males are particularly anomalous, having life expectancies at birth similar to those found among other indigenous peoples 30 or more years previously. Moreover, as we shall see in Chapter 4, there is evidence that Aboriginal life expectancy did not increase much from the early 1970s to the late 1980s.

Fourth, although Aborigines clearly have the lowest life expectancy, it is also noteworthy that American Indians have the highest, though by only a few years. This, too, deserves explanation.

Fifth, infant mortality rates have fallen dramatically in all populations. Australian Aboriginal infant mortality has dropped especially rapidly since the early 1970s, an observation to which I shall return later. Here I simply wish to point out the disjunction between the relatively low Aboriginal rates in the 1980s (ranging from 20 to 34) and their low life expectancy. In contrast, during the 1960s when Maori infant mortality was 30 per 1,000, the life expectancy (of males and females combined) was 60. I shall return to this phenomenon later in this chapter when I discuss the structure of contemporary mortality and again in Chapter 4.

Turning first to the very low levels of aboriginal expectation of life at birth, it is clear that whether or not a country is part of the British Commonwealth, whether or not it has national health insurance, and whether or not the form of

Table 2–2 Life expectancy at birth of various indigenous and nonindigenous populations, 1980s

Country or region and date	Indigenous population		Nonindigenous population	
	Male	Female	Male	Female
United States, 1980[a]	Indians and Alaska natives		Caucasian	
	67.1	75.1	70.7	78.1
Canada, 1982–85[b]	Indians			
	64.0	72.8	72.4	80.1
New Zealand, 1980–82[c]	Maoris			
	63.8	68.5	70.8	77.0
Central Australia, 1984–86[d]	Aborigines		Total population	
	52.4	65	69.3	76.4
Western New South Wales, 1984–87[e]	Aborigines		—	—
	53.5	64.8		
Australia, 1985[f]	Combined aborigines			
	54.0	61.6	72.8	79.1

[a] Indian Health Service, *Trends in Indian Health—1989. Tables* (Rockville, MD: Division of Program Statistics, Office of Planning, Evaluation and Legislation, Public Health Service, Department of Health and Human Services, 1989).

[b] Ministry of National Health and Welfare, *Health Indicators Derived from Vital Statistics for Status Indian and Canadian Populations, 1978–1986* (Ottawa: Ministry of National Health and Welfare, September 1988).

[c] E. W. Pomare and G. M. de Boer, *Hauora, Maori Standards of Health: A Study of the Years 1970–1984* (Auckland: Medical Research Council of New Zealand, Special Report Series no. 78, 1988).

[d] N. A. Khalidi, "Aboriginal mortality in central Australia, 1975–77 to 1984–86: A comparative analysis of levels and trends," Working paper no. 1 (Canberra: National Centre for Epidemiology and Population Health, Australian National University, September 1989).

[e] A. Gray and R. Hogg, "Mortality of aboriginal Australians in western New South Wales 1984–1987" (Sydney: New South Wales Department of Health, 1989).

[f] Based on aggregated 1985 data for Queensland communities, Western Australia, South Australia, and the Northern Territory, from N. Thomson, "Inequalities in aboriginal health" (M.P.H. thesis, University of Sydney, 1989), p. 39. The data on total population are from Khalidi, "Aboriginal mortality in central Australia," p. 4.

government is federal or unitary are not by themselves adequate explanations. The one striking feature that does distinguish the Australian situation from all the others is that only in Australia were there no treaties signed between the colonizing nation and the indigenous peoples.[8] The ramifications are significant, for even though treaties—perhaps like rules in general—are often made to be broken, were not signed with every American or Canadian Indian tribe, and have been honored more in the breach than in the observance, they have provided legitimacy for claims for land, reparations, and services which in their absence are difficult to make. This is particularly noteworthy in New Zealand, where the Treaty of Waitangi (1840) became the standard by which Maori claims and government responses are measured, despite the fact that the British Parliament failed to ratify it.

Why Australians did not make treaties with the Aborigines is a contentious

Table 2–3   Infant mortality rates per 1,000 live births of four indigenous populations

Decade	Canada[a] Indians	Australia[b] Aborigines	New Zealand[c] Maoris	United States[d] Indians
1950s	—	100–10 (N.T.)	57	62.7
1960s	81.5	100–10 (N.T.)	30	38.5
1970s	34.9	55 (N.T.), 79 (Qld)	21	18.7
1980s	21.8	34 (N.T.), 20 (Qld) 24.7 (W.A.)	18	9.8

[a] V. Piche and M. V. George, "Estimates of vital rates for the Canadian Indians, 1960–1970," *Demography* 10 (1973):367–82. They report a range of rates in 1970, from 20.4 in Ontario to 61.5 in the Yukon and Northwest Territory. G. Rowe and M. J. Norris, *Mortality Projections of Registered Indians, 1982 to 1996* (Ottawa: Population Projections Section, Demography Division, Statistics Canada, 1985). The 1981 rate is unadjusted for reporting errors. The adjusted figure estimated by Rowe and Norris (p. 16) is 15/1,000.

[b] Northern Territory Department of Health, *Health Indicators in the Northern Territory* (Darwin: Northern Territory Department of Health, 1986), p. 64. D. G. Hicks, *Aboriginal Morbidity and Mortality in Western Australia* (Perth: Health Department of Western Australia, 1985), p. 44; A. Gray, "Discovering determinants of Australian aboriginal population health," working paper (Canberra: National Centre for Epidemiology and Population Health, Australian National University, 1989), p. 11. N.T. = Northern Territory (15% of the aboriginal population in 1986), Qld. = Queensland (27% of the aboriginal population), W.A. = Western Australia (17% of the aboriginal population).

[c] E. W. Pomare, *Maorii Standards of Health: A Study of the 20 Year Period 1955–1975* (Auckland: Medical Research Council of New Zealand, Special Report Series no. 7, 1980); E. W. Pomare and G. de Boer, Hauora: Maori Standards of Health: A Study of the Years 1970–1984 (Auckland: Medical Research Council of New Zealand, Special Report Series no. 78, 1988).

[d] Indian Health Service, *Trends in Indian Health—1989: Tables* (Rockville, MD: Division of Program Statistics, Office of Planning, Evaluation and Legislation, Public Health Service, Department of Health and Human Services, 1989).

issue. It is difficult to argue that Anglo-Australians were more racist than Anglo-Americans. Nor can one sustain the argument that the Aborigines failed to resist the invasion and simply melted away.[9] Geddes, contrasting the Aborigines and the Maoris, noted:

> Several causes of the greater suffering of the aborigines [*sic*]. . . . In both countries the immigrant peoples were ethnically the same, but the main force of contact came in New Zealand later when humanitarian influences from England were bearing more strongly on the European residents. Secondly, the aborigines were culturally more alien to the immigrants than the Maoris. Thirdly, the type of social structure possessed by the aborigines made them less able to resist European domination and exploitation.[10]

Subsequently a number of writers have chosen to emphasize one or another of the causes suggested by Geddes. Sinclair argues that race relations are better in New Zealand than in Australia, the United States, or South Africa because "New Zealand was the only new settlement colony in the mid-century with no established settler opinion on natives to oppose that of the British government and missions."[11]

On the other hand, Howe and Fisher each contend that Maori culture and social organization made them seem to the British higher on the scale of social evolution than the Australian Aborigines were.[12] Indians in British Columbia were thought to be about midway between the other two groups. The result was that Aborigines in particular were viewed as subhuman and as having no claim on the land. Thus treaties would have been irrelevant, a view to which Reynolds has taken exception.[13] He believes that many Australians were well aware that the Aborigines had a legitimate claim to the land but that such claims, though recognized by many, were simply ignored. This is perhaps because organized warfare of the sort engaged in by both Maoris and many Northern American Indians forced the settlers to sign treaties, whereas Aboriginal resistance was at a band level and for the most part did not involve large-scale engagements.

Whatever the explanation, the consequences of having or not having treaties have been of major and continuing significance, though they differed from place to place. At a minimum it has meant a continuing but often tenuous hold on a land base. In some places this has meant little more than the creation of a rural slum without access to jobs or services. In other instances it has meant considerably more, including the provision of high-quality, comprehensive services, a topic to which I shall return. Rarely has it meant access to employment. In general, the existence of treaties has meant in Canada, the United States, and New Zealand that indigenous peoples have claims on their federal rather than their state governments.

In New Zealand, which is a unitary state, federal versus state jurisdiction is not an issue, but in the United States and Canada, Indian tribes have fought very hard to maintain their special relationship with their federal governments rather than fall under the control of provincial or state governments. In both countries as well, there have been—and continue to be—attempts by the federal governments to shed these responsibilities. Sometimes this is called self-determination for Indian tribes, but many Indian leaders think that if they acquiesce, it will more likely lead to self-termination.

Despite the obvious similarities between Canada and the United States in regard to Indian affairs—both are federal states with treaty reservations—there are significant differences between them that contribute to their different patterns of mortality decline. The Indian administration in each country has been concerned with administering Indian lands and Indian people. In the United States the latter function, the provision of health and social services, has loomed larger than it has in Canada. This seems to reflect the legacy of the greater impact of 19th-century urban reform on American than on Canadian Indian policy.

Urban reformers in late 19th-century American cities were concerned with making Americans of the masses of immigrants from Ireland and Southern and Eastern Europe and doing so by the humane provision of a variety of educational and other services. Their influence spread to the Indian Bureau as well, which assumed increasing control over services previously provided primarily by church groups. These reform policies often had untoward consequences (e.g., the Dawes Allotment Act of 1887 and the creation of boarding schools to separate children from the cultural influences of their families and communities), but they did establish the precedent for government provision of services which at a later period had more beneficial effects. In Canada, where the cities were smaller and immigration was far less massive, the urban reform movement never achieved the influence it acquired in the United States, and hence the precedent for the federal provision of health and social services to Indians was not established as firmly. These different histories continue to influence policies right down to the present.[14] For example, in the United States, health services were provided by the Bureau of Indian Affairs until 1955 when responsibility was transferred to the U.S. Public Health Service. I shall have more to say about this service later. Here I simply wish to point out the contrast with the Canadian situation, in which until the 1970s, health care for Indians was described as "second class."[15] The Canadian government has frequently denied any responsibility for the provision of health services to Indians, and only in 1979 was a policy agreed on which, among other things, affirmed the special relationship between the federal government and the Indians, including responsibility for health care.[16]

Nonetheless, as the Australian case suggests, no matter how difficult the relationship between the indigenous peoples and the federal government, from the perspective of the indigenous peoples it is still preferable to control by state governments. Having state governments assume responsibility for native affairs is not unlike using a fox to guard the chickens, for state governments have even more direct conflicts of interest over land rights than do federal governments. State governments are much more likely to be directly and powerfully influenced by local landed and mining interests than federal governments where such interests may be at least diluted by representatives of urban, reform-minded constituencies. For the same reason, state governments are much less likely than federal governments are either to be willing to provide generous health and social service benefits to indigenous peoples or to contribute to the development of community infrastructure, for indigenous people are viewed as not contributing to their tax base and as standing in the way of economic development. This was the case in Australia until the 1970s.

Writing about Australia in 1974, John Deeble commented that over the previous 20 years, low-income people in general were known to have had little or no insurance coverage.[17] In the same volume, Raphael Coolican, who had been a general practitioner in a country town for more than 20 years before the early 1970s, wrote: "In western New South Wales, the medical care of the rural Aborigines has always been the private charity of the general practitioner. Their state of health reflects the interest that the doctor and those who work with him have in the care of the poorest of the poor." He went on to observe that "most of these services are provided free. Aboriginal private patients mainly comprise pensioners, workmen injured in compensatable accidents, and car accident victims. (God bless the third-party system.)"[18]

The same situation existed in cities, as Gordon Briscoe reported when describing the circumstances that led to the establishment of the Aboriginal Medical Service in Redfern in Sydney in 1971, before the establishment of universal national health insurance:

> Because of the low levels of income of Aboriginal families, we have not yet been able to stimulate clients to join Medical Benefit Funds. While most family incomes, espe-

cially of those who work, do not qualify for the Commonwealth Subsidized Medical Scheme, the premium of the Medical Benefits Fund is too high for almost all of our clients.[19]

On the other hand, Peter Moodie felt that

lack of medical benefit was no apparent barrier to obtaining medical advice. The hidden costs of obtaining medical opinion—fares, difference between fee and sum recovered, cost of medicine—and accessability and motivation are more likely to explain the low consultation rate in the New South Wales Aboriginal group as the costs are borne by the insured and the uninsured.[20]

And, he continued, "the disadvantage is not likely to be removed through membership of a medical insurance scheme, which does not cover all the costs involved."[21]

With the constitutional change in 1967, which placed responsibility for Aboriginal affairs more firmly in the hands of the commonwealth government, and with the creation of a National Plan for Aboriginal Health in 1973 and increased support for services aimed at removing inequalities in health status, the situation began to change.[22] The available evidence suggests a significant impact on both fertility and infant mortality, as Table 2-3 indicates.[23] "The story of how this happened is simple," according to Alan Gray:

It is sufficient to take the case of only one community, and the experience related to me during a . . . survey in 1983 by a nursing sister who had first arrived there in 1967. At that time, she had been told that she should expect many Aboriginal deaths and that there was little that could be done about it. Within a year or two, a medical practitioner was paying regular visits to the community and some infant lives were being saved. For her own part, the nursing sister became responsible for maternal and child health and as increasing emphasis was put on this type of care infant deaths became less common and finally rare. The medical practitioner involved in this was also the first to introduce modern family planning technology to the community.[24]

Thus, the assumption by the Australian commonwealth government of greater responsibility for Aboriginal affairs in the early 1970s is associated with the increased availability of services and the declining infant and child mortality.

I have shown elsewhere that the provision of health care is largely responsible for the dramatic improvement in infant and child health among Navajo Indians.[25] On the face of it, this would seem to be a paradox, that in the one nation without universal provision for ensuring access to health care, the life expectancy of its indigenous people is better than in the three in which there are such programs. The paradox is only apparent, however, for it was its very absence that required the federal government to create a special federal service specifically aimed at providing preventive and curative personal and community health services for Indians on treaty reservations. Given the history of reform administrations in Indian affairs, there was essentially no other way to honor the government's treaty obligations. Indeed, the Indian Health Service of the U.S. Public Health Service is the only example of a national health service in the United States.[26]

The reason that national health insurance or even, as in New Zealand, a form of national health service would have made such an organization unlikely is that under such programs everyone has the same coverage. The object is to provide services equally across the population, and it thus becomes difficult—but not impossible—to create special services for populations with special needs. That such universalistic services can have a noticeable impact on the health of populations with special needs is attested to by the dramatic decrease in deaths from tuberculosis among Maoris in the 1950s. Ian Pool has attributed this to several causes: the introduction of free hospital care in 1938, the establishment of a comprehensive social welfare system in which the public health services were embedded, and x-ray screening of the entire population and treatment and social service support for those found to have the disease.[27] As he points out, only a state prepared to invest generously in such a range of services and necessary infrastructure could have accomplished something so dramatic. New Zealand was such a state in the decades immediately after World War II. This is unusual. More commonly in such universalistic systems, depth is sacrificed for breadth. In recent decades in New Zealand, for instance, Maoris have had to deal with a health service that has not been concerned with their unique needs,[28] and only since the early 1980s has there been evidence of greater responsiveness to Maori concerns, one result of which has been the lack of secure funding for Maori health programs.[29] Indeed, in New Zealand, where government coverage for doctors' office visits has failed to keep pace with increasing fees, the high costs of visits for primary health care would appear to be a significant deterrent to the use of such services by the poor, among whom Maoris are disproportionately represented.

In the United States the existence of a bureaucracy with skilled functionaries devoted to serving special populations, as well as their own bureaucratic survival and aggrandizement, has meant that Indian health continues to be a visible issue. Though low in the federal pecking order and not without the problems that afflict most formal organizations, the Indian Health Service has been an articulate advocate for Indians. This is all the more the case since there has been in force for more than a decade a preference for hiring Indians in both the Indian Health Service and the Bureau of Indian Affairs. Thus Indians themselves have a vested interest in perpetuating these agencies, as both providers and recipients of services.[30]

The fact that the Indian Health Service, the Bureau of Indian Affairs, and, of course, tribal programs funded completely or in part by federal monies all giving preference to Indians in employment also contributes substantially to the different employment and income patterns observed between American Indians and Australian Aborigines. On the Navajo Reservation in the 1970s, for instance, about two-thirds of employed people worked for health, education, and welfare programs, most of which were supported either directly or indirectly by federal money.[31] Thus when Indians and Aborigines are compared with the nonindigenous populations of their respective countries, Indians have a higher proportion employed than do Aborigines; a greater proportion of their income is from wages; and they have higher median incomes. That is, Indians are more nearly like non-Indian Americans in these respects than Aborigines are like non-Aboriginal Australians.[32]

Finally, attempting to incorporate indigenous and indigent people into a national health insurance scheme sometimes runs into problems such as (1) Who will pay their insurance premiums? (2) In a country that allows extra billing—as both Australia and New Zealand do—what physicians will accept such patients? and (3) How are paraprofessionals who deliver services in many remote Aboriginal communities to be paid?

In regard to the first issue, there were court cases in Canada over just who is to pay the premiums for Indians. The Indians claimed that it was the responsibility of the federal government as part of its treaty obligations. The courts stated the government is responsible only for paying for medication, not for health insurance or hospitalization (a strict reading of the so-called medicine chest clause in several treaties).[33] As noted earlier, only in 1979 was this issue resolved.

In regard to the issue of extra billing, it is clear that Aboriginal medical services can operate only where physicians are willing to work on salary or bulk bill. The experience in the United States with Medicaid (the federally subsidized, state-controlled programs for providing care to the poor) shows that many physicians refuse to accept such patients because they are not reimbursed at a sufficiently high rate to make it worth their while. A similar situation existed in remote parts of Canada where, before the passage of national health insurance, the small number of private doctors willing to treat Indians was suspected of overcharging the government for services provided.[34]

And in regard to the employment of paraprofessionals, the National Aboriginal Health Strategy Working Party observed that the Health Insurance Commission does not permit direct billing for services provided by nonphysicians.[35] Since services provided by paraprofessionals are often the only ones available, especially in remote areas, a dilemma must be resolved that has its roots in the necessity of adapting a universal system to unique situations.

Thus the timing of the decline in mortality from infectious diseases, particularly among infants and children of indigenous peoples in these four countries, is related to the ways in which different levels of government have dealt with them, as well as with the ways in which health care policies in general have evolved. The significant variables seem to be political: the degree to which services are provided and made accessible. Although culture and setting make the provision of care difficult at times, a dramatic decline in infant and child mortality can be accomplished by a health service that is adequately supported to provide both public and personal care. Such a service can have an impact on noninfectious and man-made conditions, but it cannot be as dramatic as the effects of antibiotics and vaccines, and it requires very different kinds of interventions. It is to a consideration of some of these conditions that I now turn.

THE STRUCTURE OF CONTEMPORARY MORTALITY

It has become conventional wisdom that the diseases afflicting contemporary populations in rich countries are the result of the fact that our species is well adapted to living as hunter-gatherers in small bands and is not well adapted to sedentism and the consumption of nongame animals and processed carbohydrates.[36] It has also been hypothesized that the indigenous people of the Americas and Oceania are genetically different from Europeans and are particularly susceptible to a congeries of diseases of modernization that includes most prominently obesity and diabetes but also gall bladder disease.[37] There is much to recommend this as a hypothesis to be examined, but there is also much to recommend the equally interesting fact that we are a diverse species and that the recession of infectious diseases has not left behind a residuum of noninfectious and chronic conditions that is everywhere the same. Explaining the variation among populations in these causes of mortality remains an important task. Even in regard to the four populations with which I am concerned here, the variation is large and as yet not understood. For example, as the data in Tables 2-1, 2-2, and 2-3 suggest, there seems to be a disjunction between infant mortality rates and life expectancy.

Table 2-4 shows age-adjusted rates of death due to various causes among the four populations.[38] There are several striking features. First, diseases of the circulatory system are the single most important cause of death among both Aboriginal men and Maoris. They are more significant in these two groups than they are among the nonindigenous populations of Australia and New Zealand. This pattern is just the reverse of the one observed in North America, in which Indians have substantially lower rates of death from these diseases than do non-Indians. Moreover, the rates of death from these causes are lower among Indians than they are among Maoris and Aborigines.

Second, accidents and all causes of violence follow a different pattern. They are the leading cause of death among Canadian Indians, where they occur far more frequently than they do among nonindigenous Canadians. Among Aborigines, this cluster of causes is higher than it is among non-Aboriginal Australians. It is not as high as it is in Canada, and when rates for males and females are averaged, they are about the same as the rates among American Indian males and females. Among American Indians, the rate of death from accidents and all causes of violence is lower than in Canada but roughly twice as high as it is among all races in the United States. Finally, among Maoris, these causes are of low frequency and occur at about the same rate as among non-Maori New Zealanders.

The reasons for the distribution of these two large classes of conditions, violence and circulatory diseases, are far from clear. In regard to deaths due to violence, I have argued elsewhere that the differences in rates observed among various American Indian tribes appear to be related to indigenous patterns of socialization, social organization, and social control.[39] Among band-level peoples a primary method of conflict resolution was dispersion rather than formal institutional controls or internalized self-control. When the Indians were forced

Table 2–4 Mortality rates and ratios of rates from selected causes for indigenous and nonindigenous peoples

Cause	Canada (1976)[a] Rate/1,000 Indians	Canada Ratio of rates	Australia (1984–86 or 1987)[b] Rate/1,000 Males	Australia Rate/1,000 Females	Australia Ratio of rates Males	Australia Ratio of rates Females	New Zealand[c] Rate/1,000	New Zealand Ratio of rates	United States[d] Rate/1,000	United States Ratio of rates
Circulatory diseases	1.3	0.36	4.5 / 3.7	2.2 / 0.9	4.1 / 3.2	3.3 (N.S.W.) / 1.3 (N.T.)	3.8	1.3	1.7	0.8
Accidents and violence	2.2	2.75	1.6 / 1.5	0.8 / 0.5	2.9 / 1.6	3.8 (N.S.W.) / 1.3 (N.T.)	0.6	1.1	0.4	2.3
Motor vehicle and all other accidents									0.3	2.2
Homicides									0.1	1.7
Suicides									0.1	1.2
Infectious and parasitic	0.35	3.5	0.2 / 0.5	0.3 / 0.5	9.7 / 3.1	15.0 (N.S.W.) / 4.2 (N.T.)	0.1	3.5	—	—
Neoplasms	0.6	0.4	1.2 / 0.4	0.5 / 0.9	1.7 / 0.9	1.1 (N.S.W.) / 1.3 (N.T.)	1.8	1.2	0.8	0.6

[a] A. I. Murdock, "Mortality rates in Indian and Inuit: Changes in trends in recent experience," paper no. 4 (Ottawa: Department of National Health and Welfare, Proceedings of a Workshop on Indian Demographic Trends, 1983).

[b] Data for New South Wales are from A. Gray and R. Hogg, "Mortality of Aboriginal Australians in western New South Wales 1984–1987" (Sydney: New South Wales Department of Health, 1989). Data for the Northern Territory are from N. A. Khalidi, "Aboriginal mortality in central Australia, 1975–77 to 1984–86: A comparative analysis of levels and trends," working paper no. 1 (Canberra: National Centre for Epidemiology and Population Health, Australian National University, September 1989).

[c] E. W. Pomare and G. de Boer, Hauora: Maori Standards of Health: A Study of the Years: 1970–1984 (Auckland: Medical Research Council of New Zealand, Special Report Series no. 78, 1988), p. 61.

[d] Indian Health Service, Trends in Indian Health—1989: Tables (Rockville, MD: Division of Program Statistics, Office of Planning, Evaluation and Legislation, Public Health Service, Department of Health and Human Services, 1989). p. 35. "Circulatory" includes "major cardiovascular disease": diseases of the heart, cerebrovascular disease, atherosclerosis, and hypertension.

onto reservations, this mechanism could not operate adequately. On the other hand, sedentary peoples seem to have developed patterns of social control and socialization that reduce intragroup violence, even in the reservation system.

Such an interpretation is contentious, even when the history of culture contact, deprivation, and federal policy is held roughly constant.[40] When those environmental conditions also vary, as they do in cross-national comparisons, it becomes even more contentious, not simply for methodological but also for ideological reasons. On the other hand, I believe that any explanation of these cross-national (or within-nation) differences that invokes as its sole or major variable social disorganization, stress, or deprivation is likely to prove largely inadequate. The reason is that it would lead to making assessments of relative levels of stress (or disorganization or deprivation) among societies without having any independent measures of these variables. That such an effort would lead to circular reasoning should be clear.

In regard to circulatory diseases, which have been widely observed to account for most of the excess mortality among Aboriginal men, what makes this pattern unusual is that the condition of most significance is ischemic heart disease. Table 2-5 gives the mortality rates for this condition in several populations.

The rate for Aboriginal men is eight times higher than for Navajo men and at least two times higher than for men from several Indian tribes in New Mexico.[41] What makes the Aboriginal situation even more unusual is the high deathrate at young ages. Indeed, it is this condition that accounts for the anomalous disjunction between infant mortality and life expectancy that I have commented on previously. For example, among Aborigines dying of ischemic heart disease in 1979–83 in the Northern Territory (where the rate is not unusually high compared with that for the non-Aboriginal population), the median age at death of

Table 2–5 Mortality rates from ischemic heart disease

Population	Males		Females	
	Rate/1,000	Ratio of rates	Rate/1,000	Ratio of rates
Aborigines[a]	3.33	4.1	1.45	3.33
Aborigines[b]	1.6	1.8	0.89	1.9
Navajo Indians[c]	0.2	0.05	0.05	0.02
New Mexico Indians[d]	0.76	0.21	0.28	0.15

[a]L. Smith, N. Thomson, and A. Gray, *Aboriginal Mortality in New South Wales Country Regions, 1980–1981* (Sydney: State Health Publication no. (I.D.S.) 83-169, Department of Health, 1983), p. 48. The comparison population is the population of New South Wales.

[b]M. Honari, "Causes of Aboriginal mortality," in A. Gray, ed., *A Matter of Life and Death: Contemporary Aboriginal Mortality* (Canberra: Aboriginal Studies Press, 1990), p. 140. The data refer to Queensland Aboriginal communities, Western Australia, South Australia, and the Northern Territory in 1985. These data are discussed further in Chapter 4.

[c]S. J. Kunitz, *Disease Change and the Role of Medicine: The Navajo Experience* (Berkeley and Los Angeles: University of California Press, 1983), p. 98. The data are average annual crude rates for the years 1972 to 1978. The comparison population is the white population of the United States.

[d]T. M. Becker, C. Wiggins, C. R. Key, and J. M. Samet, "Ischemic heart disease mortality in Hispanics, American Indians, and non-Hispanic Whites in New Mexico, 1958–1982," *Circulation* 78 (1988):302–9. The comparison population is non-Hispanic whites in New Mexico, who have lower rates of death from ischemic heart disease than does the white population of the entire United States (ratio of rates in 1978–82: men, 0.65; women, 0.59).

men was between 45 and 50, and among women, between 55 and 60.[42] Among Navajo Indians the median age at death in the 1970s was between 60 and 64 for men and between 70 and 74 for women.[43] And among Maoris, as far as can be determined from the published data, the median age at death for men was somewhere in the late 50s or early 60s, and for women, above 65.[44] Imprecise as these figures are, they do suggest that Aboriginal men and women die of ischemic heart disease 10 or 15 years earlier than do men and women in other indigenous populations.

When life expectancy is in the early 50s, the usual experience is that the causes of death of major significance are infectious diseases of childhood. That this is not the case, that ischemic heart disease accounts for such a high proportion of deaths in a population with such a low life expectancy, is truly anomalous. So much so, indeed, that one might question the validity of the death certification. The high prevalence and early age at onset of ischemic heart diseases are confirmed by field studies, however. For example, Edwards and colleagues observed that ECG evidence of ischemic heart disease (both "probable" and "suspect") was higher among Aborigines than white Australians, that this was true at every age starting in the 20s, and that the prevalence of ischemic heart disease increased from rural to urban aboriginal populations.[45] The relevant data are shown in Table 2-6.

Table 2-6 also includes roughly comparable data from studies of Pima Indians living near Phoenix, Arizona, and of Maoris. In each case, data from comparable studies of samples of the white population of each country are also displayed. Comparisons among countries are not appropriate because the studies all were done somewhat differently; comparisons between races within each country are appropriate, however. The results support the analyses of mortality reported in Tables 2-4 and 2-5: Aborigines and Maoris have higher rates of coronary heart disease than do the white populations of their countries, whereas Southwestern American Indians have lower rates of coronary heart disease than do white Americans.[46]

These data assume added significance for several reasons. The Pimas are often pointed to as one of those populations that exemplifies most dramatically the deleterious health consequences of "modernization," for they have a very high proportion of obese people and perhaps the highest prevalence of non-insulin-dependent diabetes in the world. (In the sample of 701 adults examined in the study just cited, the prevalence was 45 percent.) Since this condition has been said to be either a risk factor for ischemic heart disease[47] or with ischemic heart disease an effect of a common cause,[48] their disjunction in this population is of considerable interest and importance. On the other hand, the Pimas on average had serum cholesterol levels within the normal range. In general, Southwestern American Indians have lower cholesterol levels than do age- and weight-matched whites; the levels rise very little with age; and they have higher ratios of HDL to LDL compared with non-Indian controls. Moreover, they either rarely smoke or smoke heavily. They do have higher rates of hypertension than whites do, however.[49] By way of comparison, Aborigines experience higher rates of obesity, hypertension, diabetes, smoking, elevated cholesterol levels, and lower HDL to

Table 2–6 The prevalence of ischemic heart disease in selected indigenous and nonindigenous populations, 1960s and 1970s

Population	Age	Prevalence (in %)		
		Probable	Suspect	Total
Aborigines[a]	40–59	12	13	
N = 522	>60	25	10	
Bussleton (white Australians)[b]	40–59	4	2	
N = 3,410	>60	10	7	
Pima Indians[c]	>40			1.6
N = 701				
Tecumseh, Michigan (white Americans)[d]	>40			2.9
N = 8,641				
Maoris[e]	35–74	Females		16.1
N = 755		Males		7.3
Carterton (white New Zealanders)[f]	35–74			
N = 432		Females		11.5
		Males		6.5

[a]F. M. Edwards et al., "Blood pressure and electrocardiographic findings in the South Australian Aborigines," *Australian New Zealand Medicine* 6 (1976):197–205.

[b]T. A. Welbom et al., "The prevalence of coronary heart disease and associated factors in an Australian rural community," *American Journal of Epidemiology* 89 (1969):521–36.

[c]J. A. Ingelfinger et al., "Coronary heart disease in Pima Indians," *Diabetes* 25 (1976):561–65. Pima Indians live on a reservation adjacent to the major metropolitan area of Phoenix, Arizona, in the southwestern United States.

[d]F. H. Epstein et al., "Prevalence of chronic diseases and distribution of selected physiologic variables in a total community, Tecumseh, Michigan," *American Journal of Epidemiology* 81 (1965):307–22. Tecumseh is a small city with a rural fringe in the northern Midwest of the United States.

[e]R. Beaglehole et al., "Prevalence of coronary heart disease in samples of New Zealand Maoris and Pakehas," *New Zealand Medical Journal* 546 (1975):119–22.

[f]I. A. M. Prior et al., "The Carterton study," *New Zealand Medical Journal* 68 (1968):150–52. Carterton is a rural community.

LDL ratios than do non-Aboriginal Australians. This is the case particularly among those living in urban areas and/or with access to store-bought foods.

The available evidence suggests that ischemic heart disease and its known risk factors (increased serum cholesterol, obesity, diabetes, smoking, and hypertension) are relatively new among Aborigines.[50] But the same is true of American Indians. For example, non-insulin-dependent diabetes, obesity, and hypertension are widely agreed to be new phenomena that have emerged only since the late 1940s, yet there is no evidence that American Indians have ever experienced the rapid increase to such high levels of ischemic heart disease that has characterized the Aboriginal experience over the past two decades. Indeed, judging by data from the New Mexico Indian population, the rates have been remarkably stable since the late 1950s, even falling beginning in the early 1970s (slightly behind the decline in rates nationally).[51]

On the other hand, there is suggestive evidence that Polynesians may have experienced a rapid increase in ischemic heart disease along with "Westernization" similar to that experienced by Aborigines at present. Data from Hawaii indicate a very rapid rise among Hawaiians compared with all races in deaths due to arteriosclerotic heart disease, beginning in the 1920s and reaching a peak in the 1960s. In 1960 the age-standardized deathrate was 2.8 per 1,000, compared with about 1.4 for part-Hawaiians and 1.25 for all races. Since then the rates have declined significantly, as they have in many parts of the world, to about 2 per 1,000.[52] Likewise, as the data in Table 2-7 indicate, the age-specific rates of death from coronary artery diseases are higher among young Maoris than among non-Maori New Zealanders of the same age. Only after age 65 do the rates become equal.

Among Polynesians, as among the other peoples I have described, there is no constant relationship between the common risk factors and coronary heart disease. For example, among Maoris, serum cholesterol and smoking do not seem to predict the onset of coronary heart disease.[53] The relationships are even more confusing when Polynesians from several different island populations are compared, for although the degree of "Westernization" is associated with an increased risk of death, the importance of risk factors such as elevated blood pressure, serum cholesterol, and body mass index varies among them in as yet unexplained ways.[54]

These observations suggest that the generalizations about changes in diet and other aspects of life are, broadly speaking, true. It is in fact the case that with the recession of infectious diseases and with a change from rural to urban ways of life, a cluster of related metabolic and circulatory conditions have emerged that are largely resistant to interventions by providers of curative (but not necessarily preventive) health services. On the other hand, there is also suggestive evidence of significant differences among indigenous peoples that may be the result of genetic differences, perhaps having to do with lipid metabolism and/or psychosocial differences.

Table 2–7 Mortality from coronary heart disease among Maoris, 1980–84

Age	Rate/1,000 (male and female)	Ratio of rates
15–44	0.3	2.2
45–64	3.8	1.4
≥65	18.3	1.1

Source: E. W. Pomare and G. de Boer, *Hauora: Maori Standards of Health: A Study of the Years 1970–1984* (Auckland: Medical Research Council of New Zealand, Special Report Series no. 78, 1988).

DISCUSSION

It is widely agreed that the worldwide decline of mortality over the past several centuries has been the result of the recession of infectious diseases. The effect is most obvious among infants, children, and women. The relative importance of public and personal health services, social change, and economic development in contributing to this epidemiologic transformation has been the subject of much debate. It is an important debate because major policy decisions may be influenced by its outcome.

Different populations have followed different paths through this transition, depending on historical period, ecological setting, social organization, and a wide variety of other circumstances and conditions. There is no doubt, however, that health care, both preventive and curative, can have a profound impact on a people's health, even in the absence of significant economic improvement. The experiences of several of the peoples I have described in this chapter support that position, for their economic status as residents of internal colonies where unemployment continues to be high has not changed substantially over the past several decades.

Having said that health care can make a substantial different in reducing the incidence of infectious diseases, it is reasonable to ask how such care is most appropriately provided. This is an important issue worldwide, and the answer will probably differ depending on the population, not simply the culture and economy of the people, but their levels and causes of mortality as well. I have suggested that national health insurance is not the most appropriate way to provide services in populations where there are great distinctions in health needs. Private insurance would be even less appropriate. Nonetheless, the governments in many developing countries are being urged by the World Bank to follow this path, although with the specific acknowledgment that the rural poor will likely continue to need services best provided directly by the government.[55]

There are several reasons that health insurance, whether public or private, is probably not the most effective way to provide services to particularly deprived populations. First, as I have already suggested, in a society with great extremes of wealth and health, the common denominator of covered services will not be as much as the richest want or the poorest need. For instance, such health services are likely to be narrowly construed, and they are unlikely to include community development or interventions that reach beyond individual patients or, at most, coresident members of the same family.

Second, where there are great discrepancies in wealth and cultural values, the poorest are likely to feel inhibited from using services meant for all. I have noted that this has been offered as part of the explanation of the underutilization of services even by Aborigines who were covered by insurance benefits, and the same is said to be true of Maoris in New Zealand.[56]

Third, two principles of insurance are that (1) it protects against risk, not certainty, and (2) the events should be independent of one another. Thus, if it is certain that every house in a city will be destroyed by fire, fire insurance will be prohibitively expensive, and so one would be better advised to create a program supported by general revenues to provide disaster relief when the worst happens. Conversely, if the risk of being injured in an auto accident is small but the costs are very high, insuring against the risk of such an event makes a great deal of sense. Likewise, infectious diseases occurring as part of an epidemic are not independent events and are thus bad insurance risks, but myocardial infarctions and other chronic diseases are more likely to be independent and may thus be good targets for insurance.

The relevance to the epidemiologic transition is clear, for morbidity and mortality in pretransition populations are closer to being epidemic certainties than independent rarities. Programs designed to prevent or treat such conditions across the entire population therefore make a good deal of sense. As health improves and the risk of falling ill and dying prematurely declines significantly, protection with universal insurance coverage becomes more feasible, though there may be political and cultural reasons that it would still not be desirable. For example, in labor-surplus communities, work in the service sector supported by government funds is one of the few sources of steady cash income, as is the case on American Indian reservations. Moreover, indigenous peoples may wish to maintain their own exclusive services as a means of resisting cultural assimilation and the loss of whatever political autonomy they have managed to acquire. This exemplifies, as do many of the issues raised in this chapter, a problem with which nation-states have been grappling, with only partial success, for at least two centuries. That is, how are peoples who conceive of themselves as corporate groups, with cultures based on their own kinship and religious systems and with deep attachments to particular places, to be incorporated into states for which the unfettered individual is the relevant unit?

Finally, although health services have had an immense impact on infectious diseases, their impact on man-made and noninfectious conditions is more problematic. The reason is, of course, that circulatory diseases, neoplasms, and accidents, and violence cannot be prevented with vaccines or cured with anything analogous to antibiotics. The discussion of ischemic heart disease was meant to illustrate both the enormous variability among peoples and the fact that there is much we do not understand about the causes of this and related conditions. The fact that the usual risk factors do not seem to explain the differences between American Indians and Aborigines suggests that at some level the risk factors need to be distinguished from the causes. This is not to say that reducing obesity, smoking, hypertension, and serum cholesterol is unlikely to beneficial; it is only to say that in themselves they are not adequate explanations of the patterns we observe.

The variability in noninfectious diseases among peoples with similar locations in the social structures of what appear to be similar nation-states is important. Differences in health services do not seem to account for these differences in noninfectious diseases. We are thus left with an important and as yet unsolved puzzle concerning etiology. For our present purposes, however, it suffices to observe that historical and social structural similarities among peoples do not ensure that their disease patterns will always necessarily be the same. Just as diverse forces conspired to shape the various trajectories of mortality decline in the past, so does diversity characterize the structure of mortality in the present.

NOTES

1. G. Manuel and M. Posluns, *The Fourth World: An Indian Reality* (Toronto: Collier-Macmillan, 1974); N. Dyck, ed., *Indigenous Peoples and the Nation-State: Fourth World Politics in Canada, Australia, and Norway* (Newfoundland: Social and Economic Papers no. 14, Institute for Social and Economic Research, Memorial University of Newfoundland, St. John's, Canada, 1985); G. L. Gold, ed., *Minorities and Mother Country Imagery* (Newfoundland: Social and Economic Papers no. 13, Institute of Social and Economic Research, Memorial University of Newfoundland, St. John's, Canada, 1984); J. Linnekin and L. Poyer, eds., *Cultural Identity and Ethnicity in the Pacific* (Honolulu: University of Hawaii Press, 1990).

2. A. Crosby, *Ecological Imperialism* (Cambridge: Cambridge University Press, 1986).

3. I do not include other Pacific states here because they are discussed in the following chapter.

4. L. Hartz, *The Founding of New Societies* (New York: Harcourt Brace & World, 1964).

5. K. Sinclair, "Why are race relations in New Zealand better than in South Africa, South Australia or South Dakota?" *New Zealand Journal of History* 5 (1971): 121–27.

6. P. Ehrensaft and W. Armstrong, "Dominion capitalism: A first statement," *Australian and New Zealand Journal of Sociology* 14 (pt. 2) (1978): 352–63.

7. The life expectancies for New Zealand and Canada cover 14 and 6 years, respectively. Thus presenting average figures may understate life expectancy at the end of a period if the improvement was rapid. On the other hand, the infant mortality rates are for 1 year and show the same patterns as life expectancy. In addition, the definition of an indigenous person is not a simple matter. The Canadian data are for status Indians, that is, those who are defined legally as Indians. This definition has changed over time, as it has in Australia in regard to Aborigines.

8. R. M. Bienvenue, "Comparative colonial systems: The case of Canadian Indians and Australian Aborigines," *Australian–Canadian Studies: An Interdisciplinary Social Science Review* 1 (1983): 30–43.

9. R. Evans, K. Saunders, and K. Cronin, *Race Relations in Colonial Queensland* (St. Lucia: Queensland University Press, 1975).

10. W. R. Geddes, "Maori and Aborigine: A comparison of attitudes and policies," *Australian Journal of Science* 24 (1961): 222.

11. Sinclair, "Why are race relations."

12. K. R. Howe, *Race Relations in Australia and New Zealand: A Comparative Survey 1770s–1970s* (Wellington: Methuen, 1977); R. Fisher, "The impact of European settlement on the indigenous peoples of Australia, New Zealand, and British Columbia: Some comparative dimensions," *Canadian Ethnic Studies* 12 (1980): 1–14.

13. H. Reynolds, *Aboriginal Land Rights in Colonial Australia,* Occasional Lecture Series no. 1 (Canberra: National Library of Australia, 1988).

14. My discussion of the distinctions between the United States and Canada is based largely on J. Guillemin, "The politics of national integration: A comparison of United States and Canadian Indian administrations," *Social Problems* 25 (1978): 319–32.

15. T. K. Young, *Health Care and Cultural Change: The Indian Experience in the Central Subarctic* (Toronto: University of Toronto Press, 1988), p. 126.

16. Ibid., pp. 93–94.

17. J. Deeble, "Health insurance," in B. S. Hetzel, M. Dobbin, L. Lippmann, and E. Eggleston, eds., *Better Health for Aborigines?* (St. Lucia: University of Queensland Press, 1974), p. 135.

18. R. E. Coolican, "The role of the general practitioner in a rural part-Aboriginal community," in Hetzel et al., eds., *Better Health for Aborigines?* pp. 127–32.

19. G. Briscoe, "The Aboriginal medical service in Sydney," in Hetzel et al., eds., *Better Health for Aborigines?* pp. 166–70.

20. P. Moodie, *Aboriginal Health* (Canberra: Australian National University Press, 1973), p. 257.

21. Ibid., p. 262.

22. A. Gray, "Discovering determinants of Australian Aboriginal population health," working paper (Canberra: National Centre for Epidemiology and Population Health, Australian National University, 1989), p. 5.

23. Ibid., p. 10.

24. Ibid.

25. S. J. Kunitz, *Disease Change and the Role of Medicine: The Navajo Experience* (Berkeley and Los Angeles: University of California Press, 1983).

26. The Veterans Administration provides medical care to veterans and thus might be considered a national health service as well. The Indian Health Service is a true national health service, however, inasmuch as it provides public health services to entire communities as well as the full range of personal services to entire populations. Not all reservations were established by treaty. Some were established by executive order. No distinction is made between them in respect of the provision of services. Moreover, in many instances Indians resident in urban areas also qualify for services.

Provision of health services to members of federally recognized tribes derives from a long and complex history. Some treaties—for example, the Navajos' of 1868—did not include any mention of health care. Many others did. See Felix S. Cohen, *Handbook of Federal Indian Law* [1942] (Albuquerque, NM: University of New Mexico Press, 1971), pp. 243–44. In addition to treaty rights, however, the provision of health and other services derives from the Federal Government's trustee role.

> The trustee role adopted by the Federal Government has its origins in more than the United States being the technical legal owner of Indian land. Among other roles, the Federal Government was to protect tribes against non-Indians (States) and to provide necessary services. The operative documents for determining the scope of the Federal responsibility in any given situation are the treaties and statutes. In situations where the statutes or treaties are unclear, the courts have developed special rules of interpretation—rules that give the most favorable interpretation or construction to the Indian parties.

U.S. Congress, Office of Technology Assessment, *Indian Health Care*, OTA-H-290 (Washington, DC: U.S. Government Printing Office, April 1986), p. 53.

27. D. I. Pool, "Mortality trends and differentials," in *Population of New Zealand*, vol. 1, Country Monograph Series no. 12 (Bangkok: Economic and Social Commission for Asia and the Pacific, 1985), p. 234.

28. A. H. Smith and N. E. Pearce, "Determinants of differences in mortality between New Zealand Maoris and non-Maoris aged 15–64," *New Zealand Medical Journal* 97 (1984): 101–8.

29. M. H. Durie, "Implications of policy management decisions on Maori health: Contemporary issues and responses," in M. W. Raffel and N. K. Raffel, eds., *Perspec-

tives on Health Policy: Australia, New Zealand, United States (New York: Wiley, 1987), p. 204.

30. In this regard, it is not accidental that data on Aboriginal health are very hard to find; that data on American Indians and Maoris are plentiful; and that data on Canadian Indians are intermediate in completeness of coverage. Statistics are a form of advertising; their availability suggests the presence of an agency with a vested interest in publicizing the magnitude of particular problems, the agency's effectiveness in dealing with them, and the significance of the problems that still remain to be dealt with. The Indian Health Service is such an agency. Evidently the Maoris have been influential enough in New Zealand to force the health service to publicize their situation and needs as well, for they are not only an increasingly well organized population but also constitute 11 or 12 percent of the New Zealand population in a relatively small area. The other indigenous peoples are a much smaller proportion of their national populations and are much more scattered over vast areas.

31. S. J. Kunitz, "Underdevelopment and social services on the Navajo Reservation," *Human Organization* 36 (1977): 398–404.

32. R. C. Gregory, "'The American dilemma' down under: A comparison of the economic status of U.S. Indians and blacks and Aboriginal Australians," in J. C. Altman, ed., *Aboriginal Employment Equity by the Year 2000,* Centre for Aboriginal Economic Policy Research, Australian National University, Research Monograph no. 2 (Canberra: Academy of Social Sciences in Australia, 1991), pp. 141–54.

33. P. A. Cumming and N. H. Mickenberg, *Native Rights in Canada* (Toronto: Indian–Eskimo Association of Canada in association with General Publishing, 1972), pp. 128–31.

34. Young, *Health Care and Cultural Change,* p. 109.

35. National Aboriginal Health Strategy Working Party, *A National Aboriginal Health Strategy* (Canberra, 1989), p. 41.

36. S. B. Eaton, M. Konner, and M. Shostak, "Stone agers in the fast lane: Chronic degenerative diseases in evolutionary perspective," *American Journal of Medicine* 84 (1988): 739–49.

37. J. V. Neel, "Diabetes mellitus: A 'thrifty' genotype rendered detrimental by 'progress'?" *American Journal of Human Genetics* 14 (1962): 353–62; J. V. Neel, "The thrifty genotype revisited," in J. Kobberling and R. Tattersall, eds., *The Genetics of Diabetes Mellitus* (New York: Academic Press, 1982), pp. 283–93; K. M. Weiss, R. E. Ferrell, and C. L. Hanis, "A New World syndrome of metabolic diseases with a genetic and evolutionary basis," *Yearbook of Physical Anthropology* 27 (1984): 153–78.

38. The age adjustment is to the larger nonindigenous population of each country. Since age structures do not differ substantially, this does not introduce significant error. The exception is New Zealand, where the rates have been standardized to a world population that is younger than the nonindigenous New Zealand population.

39. Kunitz, "Underdevelopment and social services"; J. E. Levy and S. J. Kunitz, "Indian reservations, anomie, and social pathologies," *Southwestern Journal of Anthropology* (now *Journal of Anthropological Research*) 27 (1971): 97–128.

40. This issue is considered in more detail in Chapter 5, which compares Navajo and Hopi Indians in the American Southwest.

41. Since the New Mexico rates are age adjusted to an older population, a direct comparison is not entirely appropriate, but the crude rates of death for Indians are almost certainly lower than the age-adjusted rates reported here.

42. A. Plante, "Aboriginal mortality in the Northern Territory, 1979–1983" (M.P.H. thesis, University of Sydney, 1988), p. 138.

43. Kunitz, "Underdevelopment and social services," p. 98.

44. E. W. Pomare and G. de Boer, *Hauora: Maori Standards of Health: A Study of the Years 1970–1984* (Auckland: Medical Research Council of New Zealand, Special Report Series no. 78, 1988), pp. 72–76.

45. F. M. Edwards, P. H. Wise, D. W. Thomas, J. B. Murchland, and R. J. Craig, "Blood pressure and electrocardiographic findings in the South Australian Aborigines," *Australian and New Zealand Journal of Medicine* 6 (1976): 197–205.

46. There is evidence that Indians on the Northern Plains of the United States have rates of coronary heart disease closer to those of white Americans than to those of Indians in the Southwest. See, for example, S. L. Hrabovsky, T. K. Welty, and J. L. Coulehan, "Acute myocardial infarction and sudden death in Sioux Indians," *Western Journal of Medicine* 150 (1989): 420–22.

47. K. O'Dea, R. M. Spargo, and P. J. Nestel, "Impact of Westernization on carbohydrate and lipid metabolism in Australian Aborigines," *Diabetologia* 22 (1982): 148–53.

48. R. J. Jarrett, "Epidemiology and public health aspects of non-insulin dependent diabetes," *Epidemologic Reviews* 11 (1989): 151–71.

49. T. M. Becker, C. Wiggins, C. R. Key, and J. M. Samet, "Ischemic heart disease mortality in Hispanics, American Indians, and non-Hispanic whites in New Mexico, 1958–1982," *Circulation* 78 (1988): 302–9.

50. See, for instance, *Urapuntja Health Service Health Survey* (Alice Springs, NT: Urapuntja Health Service Aboriginal Corporation, 1990).

51. Becker et al., "Ischemic heart disease mortality."

52. M. A. Look, *A Mortality Study of the Hawaiian People,* R&S Report no. 38, Research and Statistics Office (Honolulu: Hawaii State Department of Health, 1982).

53. R. Beaglehole, I. A. M. Prior, C. Salmond, and E. Eyles, "Coronary heart disease in Maoris: Incidence and case mortality," *New Zealand Medical Journal,* no. 618 (1978): 138–41.

54. R. Beaglehole, I. A. M. Prior, M. A. Foulkes, and E. F. Eyles, "Death in the South Pacific," *New Zealand Medical Journal,* no. 660 (1980): 375–78.

55. C. C. Griffin, "Strengthening health services in developing countries through the private sector," International Finance Corporation, discussion paper no. 4 (Washington, DC: World Bank, 1989).

56. Smith and Pearce, "Determinants of differences in mortality."

Historical and Contemporary Mortality Patterns in Polynesia

In this chapter I shall consider the impact that different patterns of European contact have had on the evolution of mortality and epidemiologic regimes in Polynesia. This is as close to an ideal place as the observational scientist can find to examine these issues, for the biological and cultural similarities among peoples scattered across thousands of miles of ocean and different island environments have been obvious to observers since the first European contact (see Figure 3-1).[1] Perhaps unique in the world, Polynesia thus lends itself to the method of controlled comparison, which is as close as the observational scientist can come to an experimental situation.[2]

The first issue I shall deal with has to do with the impact of European contact on the trajectory of indigenous populations. For more than a century there has been a conviction that the peoples of the Pacific have experienced major losses at least since the time of first European contact.[3] Some researchers contend that the decline began even before contact.[4] Explanations have varied. Epidemics introduced into virgin-soil populations by European explorers and colonists are common to virtually all of them. Declining fertility as a result of declining *joie de vivre*,[5] as a result of the disruption of traditional social organization and culture,[6] or as a result of venereal diseases has also be implicated.

More recent writers have criticized these older views. Vern Carroll called this received history a "myth" that may have been true of some atoll populations but certainly not of all.[7] Norma McArthur and Ian Pool criticized both the inadequate population data used by previous writers as well as the explanations of the causes of population decline they offered, particularly those based on various versions of psychological or psychoanalytic theory.[8] And K. R. Howe argued that the impact of European contact was not as fatal as many have said and that the notion that Pacific peoples were dying out was largely self-serving and used to justify colonial domination: Because the natives were dying anyway, the best that could be done was to smooth the deathbed pillow.[9] Indeed, this was one of the arguments used to justify the United States' annexation of Hawaii.[10] The "new" Pacific history, Howe writes, views the indigenous populations as far more resilient, resistant, and adaptive than previous observers had thought.

The second issue I shall address has to do with the problems that arise when we attempt to explain contemporary disease patterns by the degree to which

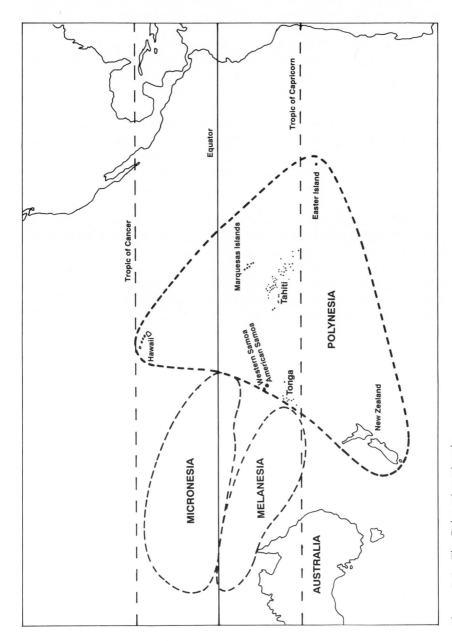

Figure 3-1 The Polynesian triangle.

people are said to be "traditional" or "modern." As illustrated in the so-called Mead/Freeman debate about Samoa, the very nature of traditional society is often far from clear and is a source of bitter disagreement.[11] The lack of clarity may result in part from differences among investigators and the periods and places they have studied, all of which have been offered as partial explanations of the different accounts of Samoan society. The lack of clarity may have to do in part with assumptions about the course and definition of "modernization" and with how we understand the persistence of what appear to be traditional forms of social organization and cultural values and their relevance to health and well-being.

The third issue has to do with how similar social structural arrangements may lead to different endpoints. I shall consider the differences in contemporary life expectancies of Maoris and Native Hawaiians to make the point that even in the so-called Fourth World of indigenous peoples overwhelmed by European contact, there continue to be important distinctions that influence rates of mortality. The fourth issue has to do with the different ways in which very different social and economic arrangements may lead to the same epidemiologic endpoint.

In each instance I shall use comparisons among and within societies to show that the demographic and epidemiologic patterns that have been reported can be explained in terms of social organization, patterns of European contact, and social and economic change. I shall deal only with some of the large islands because the small atoll populations are extremely vulnerable to a wide variety of random (i.e., unexplained) influences as well as to environmental influences such as hurricanes and drought, to which the large islands are more resistant.[12]

HISTORICAL PATTERNS OF POPULATION CHANGE

Figure 3-2 gives estimates of Polynesian populations over the past two centuries from five large island groups: Hawaii, New Zealand, Tonga, Western and American Samoa combined, and Tahiti and the Marquesas in French Polynesia.[13] Figure 3-3 plots the same data on a semi-log scale in order to compare rates of change. While recognizing the very imperfect nature of the data, several points also are evident.

First, sustained population decline was not a universal phenomenon. It is widely agreed that there were major losses of the Hawaiian population beginning in the 1780s, but the actual numbers are a matter of considerable debate. Estimates of the population at contact range from 250,000 to almost a million.[14] I have used the currently more widely accepted lower figure. Warfare, epidemics, and subfecundity due to the spread of venereal diseases all have been blamed. Certainly, the rapid growth of Honolulu from a small settlement in the early 19th century would have resulted in the efficient dissemination of a variety of diseases throughout the population.[15] Likewise, the New Zealand Maori population declined from the time of first contact, but the major losses occurred after the 1840s when their contact with the Europeans intensified. Pool's estimate of the population at contact in 1769 is 100,000.[16]

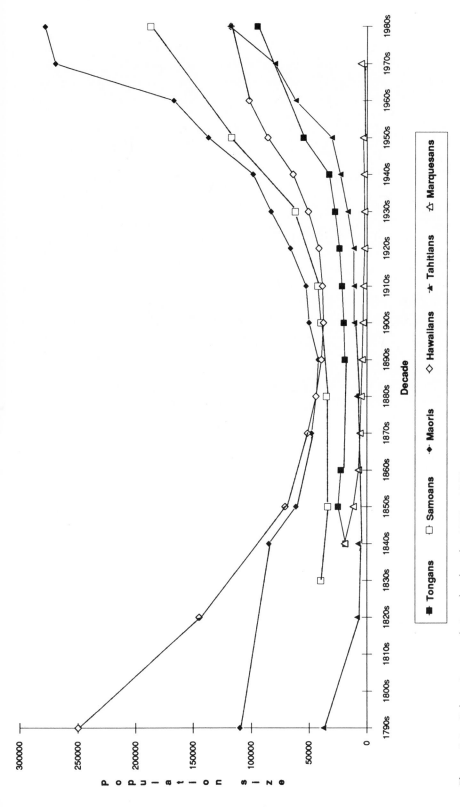

Figure 3-2 Polynesian populations by decade, 1790s–1980s

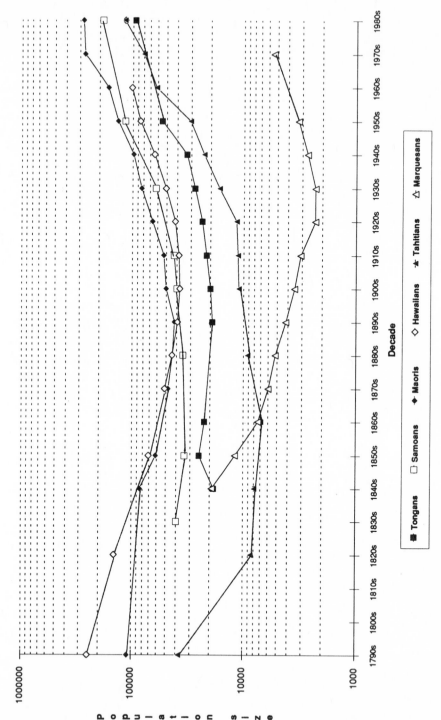

3-3 Polynesian populations by decade, 1790s–1980s, semilog plot

Legend: ■ Tongans □ Samoans ◆ Maoris ◇ Hawaiians ▲ Tahitians △ Marquesans

The population of Tahiti also fell, but the range of estimates of the contact population (8,000 to 204,000) is very large. I have used Rallu's recent estimate of 66,000 in my plots.[17] By the 1820s, however, the population appears to have stabilized. Similarly, the Marquesas lost a large part of its population, which, unlike Tahiti's decline, continued right into this century.

On the other hand, Samoa and Tonga seem to have experienced little or no decline from the first estimates in the 1830s and 1840s. It is, of course, possible that they lost population earlier, but there seems to be no evidence for this.[18] Indeed, their population trajectories in the 19th century are very similar to Tahiti's after 1820, whereas both New Zealand's and Hawaii's native populations dropped into the 1890s. No matter what their 19th-century histories were, however, all these populations but the Marquesans began to increase dramatically around the turn of the present century.

How are we to explain these patterns?

It is useful to distinguish the early period of contact in the late 18th and early 19th centuries from later periods: the second two-thirds of the 19th century, say, and the present century. In the earliest period there seems to have been a massive population loss in Hawaii, Tahiti, and the Marquesas.[19] New Zealand suffered a somewhat lower rate of loss, and Samoa and Tonga seem to have lost little or no population.

What evidence there is suggests that the intensity of contact with Europeans largely accounts for these differences. The quest for firearms provoked conflict, and their acquisition made conflict more lethal, but this was a widespread phenomenon and occurred in Samoa as well as Hawaii.[20] The frequency with which ships called seems to have varied considerably, however, and early in the 19th century was greatest in Tahiti, Hawaii, and New Zealand. On the other hand, the very large size and low population density of New Zealand would appear to have protected much of the population from contact until settlement intensified several decades later (see Table 3-1).

The more readily answerable as well as (to me) the more interesting question pertains to the differences in population patterns from about the 1830s onward. The Hawaiian, Maori, and Marquesan populations dropped, and the Samoan, Tongan, and Tahitian populations stagnated but did not fall substantially if at all. Setting aside for the moment consideration of the Marquesas, the most striking difference between Hawaii and New Zealand, on the one hand, and among the Samoas, Tonga, and Tahiti, on the other, is that during the 19th century, the former were settled by Europeans and Americans who dispossessed and demographically overwhelmed the indigenous peoples, whereas the latter became colonial outposts with a small European population attempting to extract resources from the numerically superior indigenous peoples. That is, the latter were much more nearly colonies in the usual way the term is understood. The former are examples of what Donald Denoon calls "settler capitalism," a term he applies to South Africa, Argentina, Uruguay, Chile, and Australia, as well as New Zealand.[21]

As Denoon describes it, "settler capitalism" has several characteristics that distinguish it from other versions of colonialism:[22] (1) Each began as a garrison outpost of one or another European empire. (2) "There was no dependable production, because there was no exploitable indigenous community strong enough to sustain a stratum of conquering settlers." (3) Pastoralism usually dominated production at first; then landowners consolidated control over land and labor "while a benign administration registered their titles and protected their property."[23] (4) During the 19th century "these settler societies took full advantage of new production and transport and market opportunities, to achieve a level of prosperity and a demographic and territorial expansion which none had imagined in 1814."[24] The settlers' "independence was not complete, but it was much more substantial than that which prevailed in most of the tropical world, where conquest and colonial administration prevailed."[25] (5) Yet diversification of production did not occur. Britain influenced the quantity and quality of production through market conditions rather than direct imperial control. (6) Such "unforced dependence" was the result of powerful internal forces (social classes) whose interests were compatible with British imperial interests. (7) As settler societies expanded, they came in contact with agricultural populations that, under certain circumstances, began producing cash crops and became peasantries. This was a transient phase, however, and was quickly transformed. "In general, the effect of settlers upon other rural people was to drive them swiftly towards fully capitalist relations of production, passing briskly through peasantization and plantation production merely as transitional social formations."[26]

Though not included in Denoon's analysis, much of Hawaii's history may be described in similar terms. Most significant for our purposes is the final point, that the agricultural peoples encountered by the settlers were quickly turned into wage workers, either rural or urban. This was as true of the Hawaiians as of the Maoris. In both cases, the settlers' control of land led to expropriation and the consolidation of large tracts for ranching or (in Hawaii) plantations that either employed the indigenous people or, if they could not be coaxed or coerced or were not numerous enough, imported contract labor. Similar attempts were made in what became Western Samoa and Tahiti, but for reasons to which I shall return later, such attempts were not as successful as they were in New Zealand and Hawaii.

The economic transformations of these settler societies attracted highly mobile and landless Europeans who were adaptable to the conditions of these new (to them) lands.[27] This European (and, in Hawaii, Asian) demographic wave, which numerically and economically overwhelmed the Maoris and Native Hawaiians, was partly responsible for the catastrophic population declines that each experienced. It is usually argued that exotic diseases were the cause of the decline experienced by these and other virgin-soil populations. That such diseases as influenza, measles, and tuberculosis were of enormous significance cannot be doubted. On the other hand, such diseases were also introduced into the Samoas and Tonga with serious but not cataclysmic consequences.

Others have observed that European contact in Western Polynesia (Samoa, Tonga) had less impact on the population than it did in Eastern Polynesia, although these islands were not free of exotic epidemics.[28] Pirie suggested several possible reasons: (1) Western Polynesia may have been less isolated biologically than Eastern Polynesia, so that at contact the population was less vulnerable to the Europeans' diseases. (2) Contact with Europeans may have been regulated more formally by chiefly authority in Western Polynesia than elsewhere. (3) A lower prevalence of yaws in Eastern Polynesia may have produced less cross-immunity to syphilis than may have been the case in Western Polynesia.[29]

Without disputing the possible importance of any of these factors, it seems to me most likely that social disruption caused by the kind of settler capitalism I have already described will prove a more significant part of the explanation. I am not invoking a psychosomatic explanation in which longing for the lost home results in depression, suppression of the immune response, and increased vulnerability to disease, although all of that is possible. Rather, it seems probable that the impoverishment resulting from the destruction of subsistence agriculture would have made people more susceptible to respiratory diseases and gastroenteritis, which flourish under conditions of poverty, crowding, and malnutrition. Moreover, the expropriation of land resulted in the removal and no doubt the disruption of social networks that provided both instrumental and emotional support in times of need. Observations of epidemics in virgin-soil populations suggest that social disruption is at least as significant in causing high mortality as is the virulence of the infectious agent itself, and many contemporary studies suggest an important role for social support in reducing the risk of death from a wide variety of causes. And indeed, Pool showed that during the second half of the 19th century, Maori child-to-woman ratios were lowest in those areas of New Zealand where land expropriation was proceeding most rapidly.[30]

Child-to-woman ratios are the result of both mortality and fertility patterns and thus raise the issues of infanticide and infertility as a result of venereal disease, as well as mortality due to disease and malnutrition. Infanticide, whether passive or active, has been proposed as a contributing factor in the decline of both the Maori and the native Hawaiian populations. But demographic, ethnographic, or historical research has not turned up any incontrovertible evidence, and certainly not of enough cases to have had a measurable demographic impact.[31]

The question of infertility and subfertility is less clear. There is reasonably good evidence for a decline in Maori fertility from 1769 to the mid-19th century, with some evidence based on 1844 mission records of absolute sterility among 35 percent of the women.[32] For unknown reasons, from 1850 to 1880 Maori fertility rates increased even as the population decline continued.[33]

Among native Hawaiians, too, Stannard argued that infertility due to venereal and other diseases was a major determinant of the population decline.[34] His demographic analyses are less compelling than Pool's are of the Maori data, however, and there is no way to assess the changing relative importance of mortality and fertility, as there is with the Maori data. It is true that in 1850 the child-to-woman ratio of the Hawaiian population was about as low as the Maori ratio, but this in itself does not allow one to determine the relative weights of the two processes.[35] In Hawaii as well as in New Zealand and Eastern Polynesia, premarital sexual prohibitions were less severe than in Western Polynesia, and there is evidence that this may have contributed to differences in the transmission of venereal diseases and thus perhaps to differences in prevalence rates of infertility.[36]

In contrast with the situation in Hawaii and New Zealand, in the more tropical islands the transformation of the indigenous peoples into wage workers did not occur as swiftly or as thoroughly. The traditional economy was "peasantized," to use Denoon's term. That is, the indigenous peoples engaged in both subsistence activities and the cash cropping of bananas, copra, and taro. Though attempts were made to create plantations on both Samoa and Tahiti, this never accounted for most of the suitable land or work force, as it did in Hawaii and New Zealand. It is useful to ask why.

It is unlikely that patterns of chiefly centralization and decentralization were entirely responsible. Hawaii was highly centralized under Kamehameha I at the beginning of the 19th century, but so was Tahiti under Pomare and Tonga under Taufa'ahau. New Zealand was highly decentralized, as were the Marquesas and Samoa. It is often argued that land alienation was not permitted by the Tongan king, but it is also true that Tonga was not sufficiently attractive to Europeans to make any foreign power wish to expend the effort to expropriate the land.[37]

Indeed, it is the amount of arable land that seems to account best for the differences in settlement between New Zealand and Hawaii, on the one hand, and Samoa, Tonga, and French Polynesia, on the other. Table 3-1 shows the area of each group of islands. Since all except Tonga are mountainous, the amount of land suitable for agriculture is, of course, much smaller than the total area. Unfortunately, data on the amount of suitable agricultural land are not readily available. Crocombe commented concerning land policy, "The goals of centralized [colonial] administration were to obtain effective control, reduce dispute, increase production, and *in the larger territories,* to make way for colonists" (italics added).[38] Missionaries and colonial administrators often aspired to make producers of the natives—on either their lands or plantations—and to keep out large numbers of settlers.[39] This seems to have been true on Tonga and Samoa and in French Polynesia.[40] They were more likely to succeed on islands that were not attractive to large numbers of settlers and thus where they could retain some control and therefore where massive land alienation did not occur. Moreover, in

Table 3–1   Area of selected Polynesian islands

Island(s)	Area in sq km	Population/sq km at first estimate[a]
Tonga	699	26.4 (1840s)
Western Samoa	2,934	
American Samoa	197	
Total	3,131	12.7 (1830s)
French Polynesia	3,265	
Society Islands	1,626	9.8–30.7 (1790s)
Hawaii	15,862	15.7
New Zealand	269,063	0.4

[a]See Appendix 3-1.

the few cases in which plantations were established on Samoa and Tahiti, it was difficult to get the indigenous people to work on them, for they preferred to work their own land as peasant producers.

Every bit as striking as the different patterns of decline and stability during the 19th century is the similarity in patterns of growth in the 20th century. Starting in the second and third decades of this century, there was a significant increase in all populations, again excepting the Marquesans. There is no evidence of radically improved and widespread economic well-being through the 1940s when these changes were getting under way. Nor is there yet evidence of some sort of genetic selection for disease resistance among these populations. There is, however, evidence of attempts to improve public health by the indigenous people them-selves, colonial and indigenous governments, and nongovernmental organiza-tions, particularly the Rockefeller Foundation.[41] It is not possible to assess the impact of any of these programs: One can simply point to the temporal associa-tion between such attempts and the increase in population.

First, in regard to self-help, the "Maori renaissance" of the first years of this century was a movement in which a few Maori leaders began to engage in a variety of preventive and health educational activities. Ian Pool suggested that this movement may have been responsible for, or at least contributed to, the "turnaround" in Maori mortality at this time, though firm data are lacking.[42] Another example is the development of women's committees in Samoan villages in the 1920s. These were stimulated originally by a New Zealand physician and involved influential women in each village who exercised surveillance of "child care and village health."[43] These committees continue to operate in many vil-lages, though again with effects that do not seem to have been measured.[44]

In regard to government action, quarantine was, of course, important. Just how important is illustrated by the fact that the influenza epidemic of 1918 was prevented in American Samoa, which enforced the quarantine, but killed perhaps 20 percent of the population in Western Samoa, where the new Zealand adminis-tration failed to enforce it.[45] The government of Tonga distributed free food for infants.[46] Sanitary regulations were passed by most governments, though in many places they seem to have been honored more in the breach than in the observance.[47] The protection of water supplies was attempted in a variety of places as well.

The Rockefeller Foundation's activities were originally part of the worldwide hookworm eradication campaign and also included the treatment and prevention of yaws. Because hookworm is spread by human fecal contamination of the soil, the Foundation's work on waste disposal may have reduced the spread of enteric diseases as well. As in the preceding examples, there is no way of assessing the magnitude of the impact these measures had on the mortality of the population. It seems likely, however, that the similar trajectories of population growth after the 1910s were indeed the result primarily of public health measures, which were widespread in these years.

The point I have made in this section is twofold. First the picture of population collapse painted by early writers was partly true, but not universally. It was not true of most island populations in which American and European settlement was not extensive. It was catastrophic in those populations where settlement and dispossession did occur. This is important because it suggests that the contact mediated between the new microorganisms to which people were exposed and the mortality that resulted. The experience was not everywhere the same, but the differences are largely understandable.

Even this statement needs to be qualified, however, by the experience of the population of the Marquesas, which fell throughout the 19th century and most of this century as well. Until the 1920s the Marquesans' deathrate was substantially greater than their birthrate, and life expectancy at birth was only 21.5 between 1886 and 1910, and 17.4 between 1911 and 1925, increasing to 34.5 between 1925 and 1945.[48] The same factors invoked to explain the early declines in population have been offered for the Marquesas; venereal disease as a cause of the reduced fertility, extreme maternal mortality, and high deathrates from introduced diseases, particularly tuberculosis and other respiratory conditions, and diseases of infancy.[49] What is not clear is why this situation persisted so long among the Marquesans but not elsewhere, for they were not overwhelmed and dispossessed as the Maoris and Hawaiians were. Many observers have noted, however, that violence and conflict were a continuing feature of Marquesan life long after they had ceased elsewhere in Polynesia,[50] and presumably this social disruption—thought by many to be a function of Marquesan culture itself—contributed substantially to the high rates of mortality.

From the 1880s to the 1940s, life expectancy at birth and age 10 improved more slowly in the southeastern than in the northwestern islands of the Marquesas group.[51] In 1936–45 life expectancy at birth was 49.2 years in the northwestern islands' population and 37.6 in the southeastern islands' population. By comparison, in 1944–46 the Maoris' life expectancy was 48.4, and in 1940 the native Hawaiians' life expectancy was about 52 (see Table 3-2). These data

Table 3–2 Life expectancy at birth of several Polynesian populations, circa 1980

Population	Males	Females
Western Samoa	60.6	66.1
American Samoa	67.8	75.5
Tonga	60.8	65.2
French Polynesia	60.1	64.2
New Zealand Maoris	63.8	68.5
Native Hawaiians	70.8	76.0

Sources: For Western Samoa, American Samoa, Tonga, and French Polynesia, see R. Taylor, N. D. Lewis, and S. Levy, "Societies in transition: Mortality patterns in Pacific island populations," *International Journal of Epidemiology* 18 (1989): 634–46. For New Zealand, see E. Pomare and G. de Boer, *Hauora: Maori Standards of Health: A study of the Years 1970–1984* (Auckland: Medical Research Council of New Zealand, Special Report Series no. 78, 1988). For Hawaii, see R. W. Gardner, *Life Tables by Ethnic Group for Hawaii, 1980*, R&S Report no. 47 (Honolulu: Hawaii State Department of Health, 1984).

suggest that in the southeastern islands, living conditions were significantly worse than elsewhere and that endemic diseases affected both children and adults long after they had improved elsewhere. Unfortunately, the reasons remain obscure.

My second point is that widespread population growth was recorded from the 1910s onward, again excepting the Marquesas where improvement began two or three decades later. I suggested tentatively that the most likely explanation is the fairly broad array of public health interventions introduced at this time.

The distinction between settler capitalist (or "settler colonial") and colonial society largely explains the different population trajectories of the 19th century. It does not explain the similarity of their trajectories in this century. Nonetheless, the distinction continues to be relevant in the present to the degree that the socioeconomic, cultural, and political circumstances of Maoris and native Hawaiians are similar to one another and different from the circumstances of the other populations. To explore some of these contemporary differences and similarities, I show in Table 3-2 the life expectancies at birth around 1980 for females and males in each of the populations under consideration.

In the following sections I shall use the contrast between Western Samoa and American Samoa to explore what we mean by the distinction between "traditional" and "modern" as they influence health. I shall compare New Zealand and Hawaii to explore how similar social structural situations may lead to different life expectancies. And I shall compare American Samoa and Hawaii to examine how different social policies may lead to similar life expectancies.

THE HEALTH CONSEQUENCES OF TRADITIONAL AND MODERN LIFE

It is in the work of John Cassel that ideas about the health consequences of sociocultural change first explicitly entered the field of epidemiology.[52] Drawing heavily on Robert Redfield's[53] notion of the folk–urban continuum, Cassel characterized traditional folk societies as well integrated with a coherent moral order on which all members agreed.[53] Social relationships were face to face and stable, and people were known in many different roles, not simply as occupational specialists or as family members and friends.

Cassel described modern urban society as individualistic. People know one another only in special contexts. There is pluralism of religious, ethical, and political beliefs. Values and social relationships change rapidly. Once adjusted to, he said, urban life is not necessarily stressful and damaging to health. But the transition from traditional to modern often is, because people are not equipped socially or psychologically to cope with the new situations with which they are faced.

These ideas have informed much subsequent research, including an important and valuable study of the health of Samoans to which I shall refer frequently in the following discussion. The point I wish to make is this: Notions of folk and urban, or traditional and modern, that are used to explain the higher prevalence of certain noninfectious conditions in modern societies are generally studied synchronically but are assumed to represent temporal change. The problem is that the communities that are said to be traditional do in fact depend heavily on subsistence activities similar to those practiced in past times, but the whole context in which these activities occur is so changed that to describe the villages as traditional may be misleading. The studies of the Samoans' health is a useful illustration of this problem.

I have grouped Samoa with those colonies whose history contrasts with the settler capitalist societies that developed in New Zealand and Hawaii. But of course, after 1899 there were two Samoas, American Samoa and Western Samoa, which came under the control of different colonial powers with different goals. The American government assumed control of the island of Tutuila and the Manu'a Islands, and the German government assumed control of the islands of Upolu and Savai'i.

The Americans wanted the deep-water harbor at Pago Pago on Tutuila for a mid-Pacific coaling station. The island is mountainous and not suitable for extensive agriculture, and there was no intention to turn it into a colony for the extraction of primary products. The Manu'a group 60 miles to the east was even less suitable. The U.S. Navy administered the islands with what appears to have been a relatively light hand until World War II, when large numbers of servicemen were stationed there and large numbers of Samoan men got jobs around the naval base. This was the time when wage work and cash entered the local economy on a very large scale. After the war, administration was taken over by the Department of the Interior, to which the local government is responsible.[54]

The Germans had very different goals for the two islands they acquired. They had already become the center of Germany's expanding Pacific empire. The firm of Godeffroy und Sohn, which had been in Samoa since midcentury and for which the German consul worked, acquired large tracts for plantations. In the late 19th century these assets were acquired by Deutsche Handel und Plantagen Gesellschaft, which also worked closely with the German administrator, Wilhelm Solf. Solf resisted the settlers' attempts to acquire property, believing that "German racial and economic interests as well as Samoan interests, were best served by a company-operated large-scale plantation economy."[55] New Zealand assumed control of Upolu and Savai'i during World War I. The islands gained independence as the nation of Western Samoa in 1962. These very different histories have had profound consequences for the people of the two Samoas, which may be summarized briefly.

In a study of seven villages on Tutuila in American Samoa and one on Savai'i in Western Samoa in 1986, Fitzgerald and Howard found that educational, income, and employment levels all were lower in Western Samoa and that mean household size was larger.[56] Individuals in Western and American Samoa were equally likely to get cash from family members, but the amount received was greater in American Samoa, and money was given to a wider network of kin. Though equal proportions of individuals in each place reported serving a *matai* (the chiefly head of a family), "in Western Samoa 91.7% of matai served were within the respondent's household, while in American Samoa only 23.9% were in the household."[57] This seems to reflect differences in household size but, as Fitgerald and Howard indicate, raises questions about the role of chieftainship in each place as well. Moreover, in Western Samoa, a higher proportion than in American Samoa report giving daily service to a matai (see Table 3-3).

American Samoa also has a much higher proportion of its population employed by the government and in 1990 had about as many physicians (34 providing patient care) for an estimated 46,000 people as Western Samoa did for an estimated 160,000 people.[58] Physicians were paid a great deal more in American Samoa as well. Their starting salary in 1991 was about U.S.$42,000, not a great deal by mainland American standards but considerably more than the range paid in Western Samoa: W.S.$10,785–$18,080 (approximately U.S.$5,000–9,000). The result has been the migration of eight Western Samoan physicians to American Samoa and the vacancy of a number of positions in the Western Samoan health service.[59] The same sort of labor migration occurs at all occupational levels, of course; for example, it is said that 80 percent of the cannery workers in American Samoa are from Western Samoa.

Table 3–3   Socioeconomic measures in American and Western Samoa

	American Samoa	Western Samoa
Education in yrs.[a]		
males	12.4	8.9
females	13.0	9.8
Employed in %[a]		
males	61.5	34.8
females	60.9	32.0
Mean annual income in U.S.$[a]		
males	3,256	642
females	3,969	315
Household size[a]	7.7–7.9	11.5–13.1
Residence of matai in household in %[a]	23.9	91.7
Daily service to matai in %[a]	18.4	89.6
Total population	29,301[b]	157,408[c]
Prop. pop. >15 yrs. employed by government	24.7[b]	4.2[c]
Per capita income in U.S.$ for total population	3,144[b]	712[d]

[a]M. H. Fitzgerald and A. Howard, "Aspects of social organization in three Samoan communities," *Pacific Studies* 14 (1990):31–54. Survey data are from seven villages in American Samoa and one in Western Samoa.

[b]Data are from 1980. U.S. Bureau of the Census, *Detailed Social and Economic Characteristics, American Samoa*, Report PC 80-1-C/D 56 (Washington, DC: U.S. Government Printing Office, 1984). Per capita income is from 1979.

[c]Data are for 1986. Department of Statistics, *Annual Statistical Abstract, Western Samoa*, 23rd vol. (Apia: Department of Statistics, Government of Western Samoa, 1988).

[d]J. T. O'Meara, *Samoan Planters: Tradition and Economic Development in Polynesia* (Fort Worth: Holt, Rinehart and Winston, 1990), p. 189. Data are from the early 1980s.

At the level of territory or nation, then, the story seems rather straightforward: Higher incomes and a greater availability of health services in American Samoa have resulted in a substantially greater life expectancy there than in Western Samoa. If, however, one considers not mortality rates and life expectancy but the prevalence of certain noninfectious diseases, the picture looks somewhat different. As Cassel's theory leads one to expect, their prevalence and incidence are higher in urban than in rural areas.

The conditions that have been found to increase as the infectious diseases wane are noninfectious and man-made in origin.[60] They are attributed to changes associated with "modernization," particularly changes in consumption and activity patterns and increasing psychosocial stress. I shall deal with each briefly, using non-insulin-dependent diabetes to exemplify the first and hypertension the second.

A large number of studies of non-insulin-dependent diabetes in Pacific Island populations have been done over the past two decades. They all indicate that the prevalence is higher in urban than in rural populations. Indeed, Polynesians and Micronesians, like Australian Aborigines and North American Indians, tend to have very high rates when compared with many other peoples, and it is widely thought that an as yet unknown genetic predisposition must be an important part of the explanation, along with changes in diet and excercise.

Obesity, for instance, is a well-known risk factor for non-insulin-dependent diabetes. A number of studies among Samoans show that urban residents (in the Samoas as well as in the United States and New Zealand) often become massively obese, whereas rural residents, especially men, generally do not. Part of the explanation has to do with the pattern of feasting on Sundays among both urban and rural people, unaccompanied by strenuous excercise among the urban residents to utilize the extra calories.[61] Among rural men doing agricultural work, the problem does not arise. Among women, who tend to be sedentary whether urban or rural, obesity is a common condition. But obesity alone does not explain the high prevalence of diabetes, and it has been proposed that some of the unexplained variance in the prevalence of diabetes might be the result of "stress."[62] I shall return to this issue later.

A roughly comparable but somewhat more complex picture emerges from studies of conditions that are generally thought to be stress related, particularly elevated blood pressure. Studies of blood pressure are frequent, both because blood pressure is widely thought to be responsive to psychosocial conditions and because it is easy and inexpensive to measure. Commonly, differences in pressure are analyzed and treated as an interval variable rather than normotension or hypertension being considered a dichotomous variable. The point is important because statistically significant differences in blood pressure using tests of interval data may or may not reflect differences that are of substantive (i.e., clinical) significance. Hypertension is an important risk factor for premature death, in Samoans as well as other people, whereas an elevation of 4 to 5 mm Hg may not be.[63]

John Cassel wrote that in traditional societies, hypertension is infrequent and does not increase with age, whereas in modern societies it is more frequent and does increase with age.[64] Hypertension (defined as a systolic blood pressure >160 mm Hg or a diastolic pressure >95 mm Hg) increases with age in rural and urban Samoan populations. Moreover, though the numbers are small in several of the samples, there is no consistent difference at ages 55 and above in the prevalence of hypertension across communities.[65] At ages below 55, however, there is a strong tendency for populations in rural areas to have lower prevalence rates of hypertension than populations in urban areas do. Because these are cross-sectional studies, it is impossible to know how much of the observed pattern can be accounted for by migration.

When level of blood pressure rather than a diagnosis of hypertension is considered, the data suggest that people experiencing some sort of stress have significantly higher levels. In the study under discussion, "stress is viewed as the result of a disjunction between demands of the social environment and an individual's coping resources or ability to solve problems."[66]

Assessing the contribution of psychosocial processes to increases in blood pressure is difficult because the most important determinants of elevated blood pressure are increased weight, age, and salt intake and because the definition and assessment of processes such as stress are far from straightforward, particularly cross culturally. There is, however, some suggestive evidence that occupational demands on men educationally ill equipped to meet them are associated with elevated blood pressure. Men in Pago Pago, American Samoa, with less than 7 years of education and occupying managerial positions had higher levels than did people whose positions were consistent with their education.[67] The same result is not found among women. It has also been observed that men with little education who do not express emotional complaints (on the Cornell Medical Index) have higher blood pressures than those who do, thereby suggesting—but not demonstrating—that denial of emotional difficulties may be associated with increases in blood pressure.

In a study of Samoans in California, Janes also explored the relationship between social inconsistency and blood pressure.[68] He observed that two dimensions were especially important in the Samoan community: economic status and leadership in the church or family. Outside the Samoan community he considered the same variables as had been used in the study in Pago Pago: occupational status and education (or military service). Inconsistency was said to be present when leadership roles and economic status did not match (i.e., when status was high and income was low, or vice versa) and when occupation and education did not match. In both cases the systolic blood pressures of men were significantly higher among those whose positions were inconsistent than among those whose positions were consistent. Diastolic pressures did not differ, nor were there differences among women. On the other hand, for women, problems related to family life were associated with increases in both systolic and diastolic pressures.[69] Janes wrote of his results:

> The very characteristics that make Samoan leadership status a goal that men pursue avidly are those that render its attainment a powerful stressor. Seen in this way, social inconsistency is probably as much a feature of traditional Samoan society as it is of the

stateside community. However, where wage labor and status in the wage economy become added prerequisites to the attainment of leadership status, the potential for inconsistency likely increases.[70]

This is an important observation. No studies have investigated similar relationships in rural Samoan communities where lower average blood pressures and lower rates of obesity prevail. It does suggest, as Howard argued, that the conditions of urban life are more diverse than those of rural life and that individuals' repertoires of skills and resources must be more diverse in urban communities as well.[71]

The question is whether in the Samoan context it is helpful to explain these conditions as resulting from differences in traditional and modern society. A reasonable case can be made for doing so: Rural villagers engage in activities and adhere to forms of social organization more nearly like those of their ancestors than do urban dwellers. The Samoan health study defined modernization as follows:

> Several processes of culture change are associated: increasing universality of education, commercialization and monetization, development of communication and transportation links, increasing concentrations of population, the general availability of formal health services, and the expansion of alternatives to the extended family and kin networks. In the Samoan project studies, "modernization" is used as a rubric for these co-occurring processes without implications of causality.[72]

Although it is clear that these characteristics are indeed often found together, it may be misleading to claim that if a community or population does not have these attributes, it is traditional. It may just be poor. This is an important point, for traditional implies that such communities and populations are not part of the modern world, indeed that like the mythical village of Brigadoon, they are largely untouched by it. The evidence regarding Samoan villages suggests something quite different: that agriculturalists have sought actively to participate in the cash economy and to bring improvements to their villages when they could afford them. Schoeffel observed:

> One of the ironies of modern Samoan history is that although the Samoans themselves look back upon the colonial period as one in which Samoans tenaciously opposed European cultural influences and European defined notions of economic change, the rapid pace of modernization in Western Samoa since independence suggests that colonial paternalism rather than Samoan traditionalism was the real conservative force in the past."[73]

O'Meara, in his fine-grained analysis of the economic and social life of an agricultural village in Western Samoa, supports this observation.[74] He showed that the villagers responded in the 1950s and 1960s to rising banana and cocoa prices by increasing production, selling their produce, and using the cash for such cooperative self-help projects as electrification of the village. But when commondity prices collapsed, the boom ended. "Today, lacking a viable internal source of income, they rely on external gifts. In many ways their village is more backward now [in the 1980s] than it was a generation ago."[75]

Indeed, O'Meara discovered that among the 56 village families (virtually the entire population), the single largest source of income was gifts from overseas. Of a total cash income of W.S.$120,000 during one year in the early 1980s, almost W.S.$31,000, or just over 25 percent, came from this source. The sale of coconuts—mainly in the form of copra—amounted to almost as much (W.S.$27,800). Earned income totaled W.S.$19,800; small family-run businesses brought in W.S.$14,000; the sale of taro, W.S.$13,100; and gifts from people in other villages, W.S.$11,600. He estimated that the monetary value of the agricultural produce grown in the village for domestic consumption just about equaled the income received from these sources: W.S.$120,000.[76]

There has been continuing pressure from development specialists to persuade farmers to grow more cash crops and to change the land tenure system from family to individually owned plots. O'Meara argues that the land tenure system has in fact undergone dramatic changes over the past 70 years, "yet the agricultural revolution has not followed. From this we see that traditional Samoan social institutions are not blocking development. . . . The major obstacle lies elsewhere—in the economics of village agriculture."[77]

In general, village planters have incomes lower than the Western Samoan nationwide average. Within the village, farm families earn far less than do families who receive cash from abroad, from wage work, or from small businesses. "Even among the . . . farm households, sales of agricultural products account for less than one-third of their monetary income." The income per day of labor is lower in agricultural than in nonagricultural pursuits, and the marginal return to agricultural labor is lower than in wage work as well. The economic incentives for cash cropping have been "woefully inadequate," O'Meara concluded, so villagers have turned elsewhere in their search for money.[78]

In light of these data, I should like to suggest that the continued presence of subsistence agriculture and the extended networks of kin are not simply evidence of the persistence of a traditional society and culture but are an effective adaptation to the modern world in which the collapse of commodity prices has reduced farmers' ability to participate profitably in the world market. This does not mean that the results of numerous studies showing differences in the health of rural and urban people are wrong. Rather, it means that the attribution of the causes of the differences to modernity and traditionalism may be misleading because it assumes unlinear social evolution, whereas what we may be seeing instead is two different patterns of adaptation to two different forms of colonialism and social and economic change.

The point is that there are real changes in health associated with the move from rural to urban life. Not only do the infectious diseases decline, but also some noninfectious conditions increase. Most of the increase has to do with changes in food consumption and activity; some of it has to do with changes in social organization and with the diversification of the roles that people must play. Because subsistence agriculture continues to be a viable adaptive strategy in the contemporary economic environment of rural villages, those forms of behavior and social organization that have been part of that adaptation also continue to be viable, though there is evidence of far-reaching changes as well.[79] This is not as true in cities, where the demands on individuals have become increasingly diverse and where their repertoires of psychosocial and cognitive skills must also diversify. The problem that concerns me here is the use of the labels "traditional" and "modern" to explain these differences, for they imply not simply evolutionary development from one to the other, but an ahistorical conception of the conditions under which "traditional" behaviors remain viable in the modern world.[80] It is for that reason that I have suggested that tradition and poverty have been conflated.

DISTINCTIONS IN THE FOURTH WORLD

In his 1939 monograph *Some Modern Hawaiians,* the New Zealand anthropologist Ernest Beaglehole drew a number of contrasts between Maoris and Hawaiians. Hawaiians had much less experience as farmers than Maoris had, he wrote. Of 107 Hawaiians applying for homesteads on Molokai, for instance, 12 were farmers. The rest were "stevedores, carpenters, engineers, mechanics, clerks, firemen, mail carriers, with further scattering members of professional or semiprofessional occupations."[81] Although he recognized the potential bias in the sample, he contended that the Maoris' situation was very different.

> The Maori has always been a rural people, working for himself or for the white man on farms and ranches. Once rehabilitation [the consolidation of fragmented landholdings] was initiated, the Maori, as an experienced farmer, rurally minded, well-trained in the techniques of farm life, took easily to a way of life that was merely the continuation under different conditions of an occupation with which he was familiar and at which he was well trained. By virtue of tribal discipline, enlightened native leadership and a feeling for occupational continuity, the Maori has been relatively successful where his northern Polynesian cousin, the Hawaiian, has required, and still requires, years of paternalistic support, generous financial help, and an intensive economic education before a successful citizen-farmer movement can be considered accomplished.[82]

The fact that the Hawaiian homesteaders were given inadequate agricultural land—the best having been taken by the sugar plantations—was not mentioned by Beaglehole as an important part of the problem.[83] Nonetheless, he was pointing to a real difference in the experience of the two peoples.

In regard to contemporary leadership among Hawaiians and Maoris, Beaglehole made the following observation:

> My last [Hawaiian] informant made a pertinent comparison between the lack of Hawaiian leadership and the success attained by Maori leaders in New Zealand, of which he had heard from visitors. The comparison emphasizes a valid distinction between the history and cultural attitudes of the two Polynesian peoples. The Maori tribe, the effective unit of social and political organization, never disintegrated under white pressure in any manner comparable to the breakdown of Hawaiian political

organization. Tribal loyalty is still intense and consequently tribal leadership is till respected and followed. Where leadership in modern economic schemes has passed to those whose prestige is not hereditary in the tribe, this leadership receives full support from hereditary chiefs. . . .

The disappearance of the chiefly class in Hawaii and the lack of a traditionally validated dependence of the individual upon the integrated blood group symbolized by its chief have left the modern Hawaiian leaderless at the very time when native leadership might well have formulated and pursued a vigorous policy of cultural conservation.[84]

He went on to say:

Dominant and inspired leadership on the one hand, a fiercely flaming feeling for tribal and cultural integrity on the other hand—the union of these two produced a Maori renaissance. He would be a bold observer indeed, who saw either of these two characteristics in modern Hawaii, or would prophesy their birth in the immediate or distant future.[85]

The difference in political leadership resulted from the decentralized nature of Maori social organization, which contrasted strongly with the highly centralized form that Hawaiian organization took when Kamehameha gained power after the coming of the Europeans. The intermarriage of the Hawaiian royal family with the newcomers and the loss of the land base in which chiefly status was rooted worked to create an egalitarianism that permeates contemporary Hawaiian culture.[86]

The Hawaiian and Maori experiences also reflect the differences in the economic development of New Zealand and Hawaii. As a result of the growth of the plantation system in Hawaii in the second half of the 19th century and the first several decades of this century, laborers from several different nationalities were recruited sequentially: Chinese, Japanese, Portuguese, and Filipinos most numerous among them. Native Hawaiians intermarried with all these groups to a considerable degree. Moreover, as the Hawaiians were succeeded as plantation workers by other nationalities and as the best agricultural lands were taken by the plantations, an increasing number of native Hawaiians moved to Honolulu (and later Hilo) in search of work.[87] For example, the proportion of Hawaiians and part-Hawaiians who were urban residents increased from 30.4 to 45.8 percent from 1900 to 1920.[88] The process was accelerated as jobs were lost on the plantations in the 1930s. The populations of the counties of Maui, Kauai, and Hawaii actually declined while the population of the county of Honolulu continued to increase rapidly.[89]

The residential mixing of races, though it had of course occurred in the 19th century as well, was greatly accelerated by urbanization in the 1920s and 1930s.[90] On plantations, racial groups had lived in segregated settlements. In Honolulu, ethnic neighborhoods were established, but mixing became increasingly common. "This has been most noticeably true in the case of the Hawaiians and part-Hawaiians," wrote Andrew Lind, "whose diffusion throughout the city is now unquestionably the greatest of all the ethnic groups in the city. There remains only one small section of the city where the Hawaiians and part-Hawaiians constitute the dominant group, while in 1900 one-third of all the city tracts were so characterized."[91]

The decline of ethnic or racial neighborhoods—what Lind regarded as the transition from ghetto to slum—led, he claimed, to the mixing of races, the breakdown of institutions of social control, "deculturization," and an increase in deviant behavior. "For the city as a whole we find a rough inverse correlation between social disorganization, measured in terms of juvenile delinquency and dependency, and the degree of segregation and concentration of the immigrant colony."[92] By the 1930s, then, contemporary observers were arguing that native Hawaiians had become increasingly urban, increasingly scattered among other ethnic groups, and increasingly distant from their own culture. The process continued after World War II, and by 1980 almost 80 percent of native Hawaiians lived in "urban" places (population more than 2,500), the majority in Honolulu.

In contrast, Maoris during the early decades of the century were still overwhelmingly rural, as Beaglehole's observations revealed. In 1936 about 90 percent of the Maori population lived in primarily rural counties, and it was the belief of both many Maoris and non-Maoris that they were better off there.[93] Indeed, land settlement schemes were meant to enable them to remain an agricultural population.[94] It was clear to some observers even then, however, that this would not be possible, for the population had been increasing rapidly for two generations by that time, and soon there would be neither land nor employment to support them in rural areas.[95] Urban migration was inevitable.

Indeed, in the postwar decades, Maori urban migration increased substantially. From about 9 percent in the urban areas in 1936, the proportion increased to almost 15 percent in 1945 and about 29 percent in 1961.[96] By 1986 the proportion of Maoris in urban areas (small towns and main centers) was about 80 percent.[97] Thus, although at present approximately equal proportions of Hawaiians and Maoris live in urban areas, the process of urbanization began about 40 years earlier among the former than the latter.

These differences in rates of urbanization are related to differences in the economic histories of Hawaii and New Zealand. I have already said that plantations ceased to be the single dominant force in Hawaii's economic life in the 1930s. Since World War II the tourist industry has emerged as a major employer, with Hawaiians generally working at the lowest levels of the occupational hierarchy.[98] Over the same period New Zealand's economy has also shifted from the production of agricultural goods for export to the production by protected industries of manufactured goods for the domestic market.[99] As in the case of native Hawaiians, so too in the case of Maoris, there is overrepresentation at the lower ends of the occupational and economic hierarchy.

In general the American (and Hawaiian) economy has been more ebullient than New Zealand's, though New Zealand has historically devoted a larger proportion of its resources to health and welfare benefits for its citizens. According to the World Bank, in 1986 the GNP per capita in the United States was $17,480, whereas in New Zealand it was U.S.$7,460. In Hawaii in 1983 the comparable figure was $12,100;[100] presumably it was slightly higher in 1986. I have estimated Maori per capita income in 1986 to have been about U.S.$3,600.[101] The per capita income of native Hawaiians in 1979 was $5,328.[102] These data, and particularly those for the Maoris, are not precise, nor do they give an adequate picture of the inequalities of income distribution within each group. They do, however, give a broad picture of the magnitude of the income differences between them.

These historical and contemporary differences in urbanization and income are associated with historical and contemporary mortality patterns. Table 3-4 gives data on the life expectancy at birth for most of this century for Maoris and Hawaiians, and Table 3-5 shows the average annual changes in life expectancy at birth from one decade to the next.[103]

It is clear that in the 1920s and early 1930s Maori life expectancy was greater than Hawaiian life expectancy at birth. It is also clear, however, that Maori life expectancy was essentially stagnant from the mid-1920s to the mid-1940s, whereas Hawaiian life expectancy improved substantially over the same period. Life expectancy improved dramatically in the 1940s for Hawaiians and in the 1940s and 1950s for Maoris. Improvement continued right up to the early 1980s, the last years for which data are available. Despite the dramatic improvement of Maori life expectancy since World War II, their life expectancy in 1980–82 was still substantially less than the Hawaiians'. As Table 3-6 indicates, the differences are not simply due to infant and child mortality but are evident at every age. For example, Hawaiians have a higher expectation of life at age 65 than Maoris do at age 60.

Table 3–4   Maoris' and Hawaiians' life expectancy at birth, 20th century

	Maoris[a]		Hawaiians[b]	
Date	Male	Female	Male	Female
1910	32.5		30.2	30.4
1920	N.A.	N.A.	35.9	34.2
1925–27	49.4–46.6	49.6–44.7	N.A.	N.A.
1930	N.A.	N.A.	42.2	43.7
1935–37	46.3–48.8	46.0–48.0	N.A.	N.A.
1940	N.A.	N.A.	51.0	53.8
1944–46	48.8	48.0	N.A.	N.A.
1950	54.1	55.9	61.3	64.0
1960	59.1	61.4	63.0	67.0
1970	61.0	65.0	65.0	69.9
1980	63.8	68.5	70.9	76.0

[a]For 1910, D. I. Pool, *Population of New Zealand*, vol. 1, Country Monograph Series no. 12 (Bangkok: United Nations Economic and Social Commission for Asia and the Pacific, 1985), p. 232. For 1920s to 1960s, D. I. Pool, *The Maori Population of New Zealand, 1769–1971* (Auckland: Auckland University Press, 1977), p. 154. For the 1970s to 1980s, E. Pomare and G. de boer, *Hauora: Maori Standards of Health: A Study of the Years 1970 to 1984* (Auckland: Medical Research Council of New Zealand, Special Report Series no. 78, 1988), p. 31. The figures for 1950, 1960, 1970, and 1980 for the Maoris are in reality 1950–52, 1960–62, 1970–72, and 1980–82.

[b]For 1910s to 1970s, R. W. Gardner, "Ethnic differentials in mortality in Hawaii, 1920–1970," *Hawaii Medical Journal* 39 (1980):222. Gardner writes that the figures for 1910 "should be viewed skeptically." For 1980, R. W. Gardner, *Life Tables by Ethnic Group for Hawaii, 1980*, R&S Report no. 47 (Honolulu: Hawaii State Health Department, 1984), p. 13.

Table 3–5 Maoris' and Hawaiians' average annual changes in life expectancy at birth, 20th century

Years	Maoris	Hawaiians
1920–30	N.A.	0.79
1925–27 to 1935–37	0.0	N.A.
1930–40	N.A.	0.94
1935–37 to 1944–46	0.12	N.A.
1940–50	N.A.	1.03
1944–46 to 1950–52	1.1	N.A.
1950–60	0.53	0.23
1960–70	0.28	0.25
1970–80	0.32	0.6

N.A.: Not available.
Source: Derived from Table 3–4. Females and males are combined.

There are several issues to examine. Why did Maoris have higher life expectancy than Hawaiians in the 1920s? Why did Hawaiian life expectancy accelerate between the 1920s and the 1940s when life expectancy was stagnant among Maoris, improving only in the late 1940s? What accounts for the patterns of change between the 1950s and the 1970s? And why is life expectancy at every age now greater for Hawaiians than Maoris? The answers can only be suggestive, not definitive.

In regard to the first question, Pool wrote that from the late 19th century to the

Table 3–6 New Zealand Maoris' and native Hawaiians' life expectancy at various ages, circa 1980

Age	Maoris (1980–82)[a]		Hawaiians and part-Hawaiians (1980)[b]	
	Males	Females	Males	Females
0	63.8	68.5	70.9	76.0
5	N.A.	N.A.	67.4	72.2
15	N.A.	N.A.	57.6	62.4
20	46.2	50.7	N.A.	N.A.
25	N.A.	N.A.	48.6	52.8
35	N.A.	N.A.	39.7	43.3
40	28.1	31.9	N.A.	N.A.
45	N.A.	N.A.	31.0	34.0
55	N.A.	N.A.	23.1	25.4
60	13.4	16.4	N.A.	N.A.
65	N.A.	N.A.	16.2	17.5
75	N.A.	N.A.	10.2	10.5

[a] E. Pomare and G. de Boer, *Hauora: Maori Standards of Health: A Study of the Years 1970 to 1984* (Auckland: Medical Research Council of New Zealand, Special Report Series no. 78, 1988), p. 31.
[b] R. W. Gardner, *Life Tables by Ethnic Group for Hawaii, 1980*, R&S Report no. 47 (Honolulu: Hawaii State Department of Health, 1984), p. 13.

1910s and 1920s Maori life expectancy increased dramatically at the time when "in what would today be termed a 'primary health care' programme, the Maori medical practitioners who joined the fledgling Department of Public Health attacked more immediate risk factors such as nutrition and basic hygiene, as well as some of the underlying aspects of Maori social and economic deprivation."[104] This so-called Maori renaissance may well have had a great impact on living conditions and health in the first several decades of this century. Nothing comparable occurred among native Hawaiians at that time, as Beaglehole's observations suggest. On the other hand, Maori life expectancy began to stagnate in the late 1920s while Hawaiian life expectancy continued to increase rapidly. Why?

It seems likely that the explanation has to do with the effect of the Depression on the primarily rural Maoris, which must have weakened many public health programs. Hawaiians, however, were moving in large numbers to Honolulu in these same years. Though undoubtedly creating social disruption of the sort described by Lind and others in the 1920s and 1930s, this migration occurred when urban mortality had for the first time become lower than rural mortality for people throughout Western Europe and North America. That is, by the late 19th century, public health measures were being introduced in cities and having a profound effect on the spread of communicable diseases, particularly those that were food and water borne. Immigrants to American cities from poverty-stricken parts of Eastern, Central, and Southern Europe had lower infant mortality rates than did people who remained behind.[105] There is no reason to think that the experience of urban migration would have been different for native Hawaiians.

A supporting piece of evidence comes from a comparison of changes in life expectancy at birth of the entire native Hawaiian population with those of native Hawaiians on the big island of Hawaii, which is primarily rural except for the urbanized area of Hilo (see Table 3-7). Clearly, the rate of improvement for people on the big island was substantial but much less than it was for the total native Hawaiian population.

The dramatic acceleration of Maori life expectancy after World War II cannot be adequately explained by the same kind of urbanization that influenced Hawai-

Table 3–7   Life expectancy at birth, total native Hawaiian population and native Hawaiian population of the island of Hawaii, various years

Year	Total native Hawaiian population[a]	Island of Hawaii[b]
1910	30.2	29.5
1920	35.9	31.3
1930	42.2	35.5
1940	51.0	39.2
1950	61.3	45.9

[a]Data from Table 3–4.

[b]R. K. Fleischman, *Death in Paradise: Big Island Mortality 1910–1950*, R&S Report no. 40 (Honolulu: Hawaii State Department of Health, 1982), p. 7. Figures are for 5 years centered on the census year, for example, 1910 is 1908–12.

ian life expectancy during the interwar years, for the Maoris remained predominantly rural until well into the 1960s. It seems instead to have been the result of major changes in public policy. Ian Pool summarized them as follows:

> Decreases [in mortality] were produced by a combination of factors: (a) the introduction in 1938 and extension over the next few years of a free health care scheme giving equal access to hospital and other services (before 1938 health care was on a fee-for-service basis, or by charity); (b) the slotting of this into a comprehensive social welfare system also introduced in 1938; (c) the introduction of new medical technology, notably antibiotics and chemotherapeutic drugs.[106]

The gains in Native Hawaiian life expectancy, which were almost as great as were the gains for the Maoris in the 1940s, seem to me almost certainly due to the availability of antibiotics as well as the rapid postwar expansion of the economy. There were no special programs devoted to improving the health of Hawaiians of anything like the magnitude of those for the Maoris during that time. On the other hand, increasing employment in wage work was accompanied by increasing health insurance coverage which would have facilitated access to medical care. For instance, in a study in 1967 (admittedly some years after the period of the most dramatic improvement), 86 percent of a sample of Hawaiians living in a community about an hour's drive from Honolulu had some form of health insurance coverage, compared with 70 percent of the national population at that time.[107]

For Native Hawaiians and Maoris, the rate of improvement diminished after the 1950s because of both the rapid decrease in the importance of infectious diseases as a cause of death and an increase in the incidence of noninfectious conditions such as cardiovascular diseases, cancer, and diabetes. Among the Maoris the data from the mid-1960s suggest that obesity, hypertension, diabetes, and cardiovascular diseases had become prevalent. For example, the death rate from ischemic heart disease among Maoris aged 65 and above was 140/10,000 in 1956–60[108] and 183/10,000 in 1980–84.[109] Because of the way the published data are presented, it is more difficult to detect the pattern of change for those aged 45 to 64 over this same period, but from 1975 to 1980–84, there was a decline in deaths from ischemic heart disease. Pomare noted that there had been little change from 1968 to 1975.[110] The age-specific death rate from hypertensive heart disease among Maoris aged 65 and above was essentially unchanged from 1954–58 to 1975 and then dropped from 24/10,000 to 13.2/10,000 in 1980–84. The pattern seems to have been roughly the same among people 45 to 64 years old.[111]

Although these data are made somewhat murky by changes in the accuracy of diagnosis, coding conventions, and diagnostic rubrics, there is some reason to believe that among middle-aged people, deaths from hypertensive and coronary heart disease increased through the 1960s and then began to fall in the 1970s. Indeed, the decrease in death rates from ischemic heart disease probably contributed substantially to the slight increase in the years added to life expectancy from 1970 to 1980.

A similar pattern has been observed among Native Hawaiians. Deaths due to hypertensive heart disease peaked in 1950 and have fallen continuously since then. Deaths from arteriosclerotic heart disease and diabetes peaked in the 1960s and have dropped since then.[112] The increase in the number of years added to life expectancy from 1970 to 1980 is probably due largely to these recent improvements, which parallel improvements in other populations in Western Europe, North America, New Zealand, and Australia. Thus, although there have been parallel changes in the cause-of-death structures of both populations, they seem to have been the result of somewhat different constellations of forces. Urbanization and economic improvement seem to have begun earlier for the Hawaiians and to have been relatively more important than specific health and welfare policies to improving life expectancy. The reverse seems to have been true for the Maoris.

There is some suggestive evidence that these differences may also help explain the contemporary differences in life expectancy displayed in Table 3-6. I have already shown that Hawaiians' per capita income is higher than Maoris' income. There is also evidence that the educational attainments of Hawaiians are greater than those of Maoris, perhaps because of their longer history of urban life. In 1981 the proportion of Maoris aged 15 and above who had finished the seventh form (high school) was 18.6 percent.[113] In 1980 the proportion of Native Hawaiians aged 15 and above who had graduated from high school was about 62 percent.[114] Leaving aside questions of educational quality and equivalence, the important point is that a far higher proportion of Hawaiians than Maoris had satisfied criteria that either would allow them to go on to further education or would equip them with the minimum credentials necessary for employment.

Higher income and educational attainment usually translate into improved health in a variety of ways: through the ability to purchase better housing and safer automobiles, through differences in exposure to occupational hazards, and through differences in behavior. I have not found good comparative data on all these domains, but some information is available. For example, among Maori men, the mean body mass index varies from 27.9 to 35.2, depending on age; among women, it varies between 25.8 and 30.5. Among Hawaiian males, the average body mass index is 26.6; among females, 25.4.[115] Maoris thus tend to be somewhat more obese than Hawaiians. Among Hawaiians, 43 percent of males and 38 percent of females are smokers, whereas among Maoris the comparable figures are 53.5 percent and 58.5 percent.[116] It is difficult to compare the consumption of carbohydrates, fats, and protein because of the way the data are presented. It appears, however, that the average daily intake of fats, proteins, and cholesterol is lower among Hawaiians than among Maoris and that Hawaiians' intake of saturated fats is lower and of unsaturated fats is higher than Maoris'.[117] In regard to prevalence rates of hypertension, again comparisons are very difficult, owing to problems of age adjustment and definitional criteria. But taking all that into account, the reported rates do not appear much different.[118] In each case the rates (including borderline cases) seem to be in the vicinity of 500/10,000 (age adjusted to the nonindigenous populations in each instance). Thus many—

but by no means all—of the measures that are considered risk factors for various noninfectious diseases seem to be elevated more among Maoris than Hawaiians.

Causes of death do not differ dramatically, however. For example, Table 3-8 displays the data for all forms of heart disease. The absence of similar data prevents the same sort of comparison of death rates from various cancers. Thus it is not possible using the published data to determine what causes of death are responsible for the lower life expectancy among Maoris than Hawaiians. One can say, however, that the differences in life expectancy are compatible with the differences in income, education, and risk factors reported for each population.[119]

These differences between Maoris and Native Hawaiians suggest the following: The similarity in their histories of contact has resulted in similar consequences regarding their incorporation into the lowest economic and occupational ranks of the settler societies that engulfed them. This has meant that in each society their health status and life expectancies are less favorable than those of other groups. Understandably it is these inequalities and the legacy of injustices of which they are a part that are the concern of the people themselves.

On the other hand, the two societies have had different economic histories and have pursued different social policies. The result has been that native Hawaiians are among the poorest of an affluent society, whereas Maoris are among the poorest of a middle-income society. New Zealand's social policies have ameliorated these conditions, particularly in the 1940s and 1950s when infectious diseases were predominant. In the current epidemiologic regime, dominated by noninfectious diseases, such interventions are unlikely to have as profound an effect, even if the political commitment were as vigorous as it was four decades ago. Thus the differences between these two populations support the conventional wisdom that it is better to be rich than poor, as well as the more contentious notion that generally it is better to be poor in a rich country than in a poor one. And finally, they lead us to ask, under what economic and epidemiologic conditions can social welfare policies (including but not limited to health care) overcome low income to increase a population's health to a level comparable with that of a higher-income population?

Table 3–8 Age-specific death rates/10,000 population, due to all forms of heart disease, Native Hawaiians and Maoris

Population	Males		Females	
	45–64	>65	45–64	>65
Native Hawaiians (1980–86)[a]	59.3	268.8	33.3	217.9
Maoris (1980–84)[b]	67.9	285.9	34.2	204.8

[a]E. L. Wegner, "Hypertension and heart disease," *Social Process in Hawaii* 32 (1989):125.

[b]E. Pomare and G. de Boer, *Hauora: Maori Standards of Health: A Study of the Years 1970 to 1984* (Auckland: Medical Research Council of New Zealand, Special Report Series no. 78, 1988), pp. 74–76.

SETTLER COLONIALISM AND WELFARE STATE COLONIALISM

The question with which the previous section ended may be addressed by considering how peoples with histories as different as those of the Hawaiians and American Samoans have attained such similar life expectancies. The material presented so far may be used to draw a number of contrasts between them. Clearly, their 19th-century populations' histories have been quite different: Hawaiian numbers declined dramatically; Samoan numbers remained essentially constant. Hawaiians were deprived of land; Samoans were not. Hawaiians had sexual relations and bore children with members of other races; Samoans have not done so to nearly the same extent. Native Hawaiians and part-Hawaiians have tended to remain in Hawaii; a very high proportion of Samoans have emigrated. Per capita income in 1979 was $5,328 for Hawaiians and $3,144 for Samoans in American Samoa. The proportion of people 15 years of age and older who were high school graduates in 1980 was 62 percent among Hawaiians and 40 percent among American Samoans. The proportion of people 15 years of age and above in the labor force was 63.4 percent among Hawaiians and 45.5 percent among American Samoans, and of these, 24 percent and 50 percent, respectively, were employed by a government agency.[120] Thus, unemployment is higher in American Samoa than among Hawaiians in Hawaii, and a higher proportion of the employment that does exist is with the government.

American Samoa is among the most extreme examples of what have been called MIRAB states. This is an acronym that has been applied to Pacific island microstates characterized by high levels of migration, remittances from abroad, foreign aid, and bureaucracy.[121] Aid is provided by the former colonial powers for either strategic or ethical reasons. The term "welfare state colonialism" has been applied to this relationship, for the island microstates are clearly dependent on the former colonial powers, but just as clearly the situation is different from simple colonialism. In this context, aid may be regarded as a form of rental income. Since it is not a loan, it does not have to be repaid, and therefore it does not lead to indebtedness. Although often given for economic development, such funds in fact largely finance local government. Thus government jobs are attractive because they are stable and the major local source of cash income in many of these island economies. As my discussion of Western Samoa illustrated, the other major source of cash is remittances from kinfolk working abroad.

These patterns also characterize Indian reservations in the United States. Rather than strategic concerns, aid is provided to meet treaty obligations. And indeed, American Samoa is similar to an Indian reservation. It is administered by the same federal agency (the Department of the Interior); it has the same service-based employment and economic structure; and it has a similar health care system, with services generally being accessible and provided at little or no cost to the patient.[122]

If American Samoa is like an Indian reservation, however, the situation of native Hawaiians is much like that of American Indians east of the Mississippi. These tribes were conquered during the colonial period, and therefore when treaties were made, it was not with the federal government but with the governments of the original colonies, which subsequently became states. State governments have not honored their treaty obligations as has the federal government because they are under much more undiluted pressure from mining, ranching, forestry, and (in Hawaii) plantation and tourist industry interests to allow the natives' land to be used for the profit of others. Countervailing pressures from reform-minded urban constituencies are more likely to be able to influence the federal government than the state governments. Thus, like Indians in the eastern United States, Native Hawaiians are much more integrated into the nonindigenous population than are Indians on federal reservations or than American Samoans. Also like Indians in the eastern United States, Native Hawaiians are attempting to gain recognition by the federal government of a special status that would entitle them to many of the same benefits enjoyed by American Samoans and Indians on federal reservations: the return of land; access to special health services, special schools and educational programs; and so on.[123] This may be seen as an attempt to convert the dispossession characteristic of settler colonialism into the entitlements characteristic of welfare state colonialism.

These different patterns of colonial contact have, however, resulted in rather similar life expectancies at present. The fact that the per capita income in American Samoa is about 60 percent of the per capita income of Native Hawaiians and roughly the same as that of Maoris suggests that it is their stable if low level of employment, the safety valve of emigration, and the high level of services (including not simply personal care but public health programs as well) that is largely responsible for the similarities. A comparison of the survival curves (see Figure 3-4) and infant mortality rates for 1980 indicate that the slightly lower life expectancy at birth of American Samoan than Hawaiian men was the result of somewhat higher deathrates at all ages, particularly in adulthood. The life expectancy of women in each population was essentially the same.[124]

The contrast between Maoris and Native Hawaiians suggests that a reasonably buoyant economy such as Hawaii's could lead to increases in life expectancy even in the absence of special entitlement programs and that a depressed economy such as New Zealand's, in which such programs were eroding, would produce comparatively less favorable life expectancies. The contrast between Hawaiians and American Samoans suggests that generous welfare entitlements can in fact lead to high life expectancy even in the absence of a buoyant economy. Such a result may seem obvious. It is not. If it were, there would be far less disagreement about the health consequences of such programs, although disagreement would certainly persist over their economic viability, especially if they are universalized.

CONCLUSIONS

Several points emerge from the preceding discussion. They have to do with biologic, social, and economic determinism. By biologic determinism I mean the argument put forth by several historians, most notably perhaps William McNeil and Alfred Crosby, and in more popular form by Alan Moorehead, that the impact of European contact on the peoples of the Americas and Oceania was uniformly

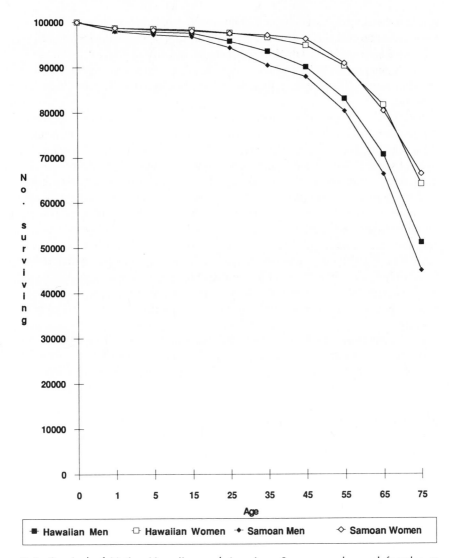

3-4 Survival of Native Hawaiian and American Samoan males and females at various ages, 1980

cataclysmic in regard to population size.[125] To deny that contact led to widespread population decline is as unreasonable as denying that the Holocaust took place. Nonetheless, it is now clear that there were differences in the responses of virgin-soil populations to newly introduced diseases. Not all succumbed in large numbers. The kind of colonial contact that occurred was of enormous importance. The significance of this observation is that it means that social forces mediated between newly introduced infectious organisms and their human hosts.

Lest we be tempted to conclude, however, that social forces are all-important and that the science-based control of infectious diseases is largely irrelevant—what I have termed social determinism—the history of simultaneous population increase across societies with different histories of colonial contact should prove a useful antidote. To be sure, these public health interventions were themselves social products. Nonetheless, they were broadly effective in several different contexts.

Finally, the recent history of these various societies indicates that economic development is not invariably associated with high life chances and nondevelopment with low life chances. The relatively high life expectancies of the populations of some MIRAB states and Indian reservations suggests that heavily subsidized nondevelopment may be an equally effective way to improve the health and well-being of certain peoples: those whose lands are too remote, too small, and too poor in natural resources to ever be truly "developed." This, of course, means a transfer of wealth from rich to poor, and it is thus only in special cases—for example, for strategic considerations, as a result of treaty obligations, or for other historically unique reasons—that the rich nations have been willing (often reluctantly) to provide such aid at a relatively high level and on a continuing basis. Nonetheless, the existence of such cases does suggest that throwing money at a problem can in some important instances ameliorate it, even if not solve it entirely.

Polynesia, then, provides an unparalleled opportunity to examine the health consequences of European contact over a period of two centuries. The historical picture has turned out to be complex: neither as uniformly catastrophic as older interpretations had it nor as benign as the new Pacific history suggests. Similarly, the recent past and the present are surprisingly complex as well. For all its undoubted injustices, economic growth has led to unrivaled improvements in life expectancy in Hawaii. But so has economic nondevelopment in certain circumstances. Biological, social, or economic theories alone cannot adequately explain the evolution of population and mortality over the past 200 years.

NOTES

1. There is some reason to believe that there may be more diversity in the biological inheritance of Polynesians than is commonly assumed, an issue beyond the bounds of this chapter. See R. Langdon, *The Lost Caravel Re-explored* (Canberra: Brolga Press, 1988).

2. F. Eggan, "Social anthropology and the method of controlled comparison," *American Anthropologist* 56 (1954): 743–63; D. Oliver, *Two Tahitian Villages: A Study in Comparison* (Laie, HI: Institute for Polynesian Studies, Brigham Young University, Hawaii Campus, 1981).

3. W. H. R. Rivers, ed., *Essays on the Depopulation of Melanesia* (Cambridge: Cambridge University Press, 1922); S. M. Lambert, *The Depopulation of Pacific Races,* Bernice P. Bishop Museum Special Publication no. 23 (Honolulu: Bernice P. Bishop Museum 1934); H. Hamlin, "The problem of the depopulation in Melanesia," *Yale Journal of Biology and Medicine* 4 (1932): 301–21.

4. S. H. Roberts, *Population Problems in the Pacific* (London: George Routledge and Sons, 1927).

5. Rivers, *Essays*.

6. G. H. L.-F. Pitt-Rivers, *The Clash of Culture and the Contact of Races* (London: George Routledge and Sons, 1927).

7. V. Carroll, "The population of Nukuoro in historical perspective," in V. Carroll, ed., *Pacific Atoll Populations* (Honolulu: University of Hawaii Press, 1975), pp. 344–416.

8. N. McArthur, *Island Populations of the Pacific* (Canberra: Australian National University Press, 1968); D. I. Pool, *The Maori Population of New Zealand, 1769–1971* (Auckland: Auckland University Press, 1977).

9. K. R. Howe, *Where the Waves Fall* (Honolulu: University of Hawaii Press, 1984), pp. 347–52.

10. L. Heffernan, "From independent nation to client state: The metamorphosis of the Kingdom of Hawai'i in the pages of the North American Review in the nineteenth century," *Hawaiian Journal of History* 22 (1988): 223.

11. M. Mead, *Coming of Age in Samoa* (New York: Morrow, 1928); M. Mead, *Social Organization of Manu'a* (Honolulu: Bernice P. Bishop Museum, 1930); D. Freeman, *Margaret Mead and Samoa: The Making and Unmaking of an Anthropological Myth* (Cambridge, MA: Harvard University Press, 1983); L. D. Holmes, *Quest for the Real Samoa: The Mead/Freeman Controversy and Beyond* (South Hadley, MA: Bergin and Garvey, 1987); L. D. Holmes and E. R. Holmes, *Samoan Village Then and Now* (Fort Worth: Harcourt Brace Jovanovich, 1992).

12. A. Vayda, "Polynesian cultural distributions in new perspective," *American Anthropologist* 61 (1959): 817–28; N. McArthur, I. W. Saunders, and R. L. Tweedie, "Small population isolates: A microsimulation study," *Journal of the Polynesian Society* 85 (1976): 307–26.

13. Appendix 3-1 contains the numbers on which the figure is based as well as the sources from which they are taken. All the sources are secondary; that is, I have used estimates made by contemporary historical demographers who themselves have analyzed the primary data.

14. R. C. Schmitt, *Demographic Statistics of Hawaii, 1778–1965* (Honolulu: University of Hawaii Press, 1968); D. Stannard, *Before the Horror: The Population of Hawai'i on the Eve of Western Contact* (Honolulu: Social Science Research Institute, University of Hawaii, 1989); E. D. Nordyke, *The Peopling of Hawaii* (Honolulu: University of Hawaii Press, 1989).

15. G. Daws, "Honolulu in the 19th century: Notes on the emergence of urban society in Hawaii," *Journal of Pacific History* 2 (1967): 77–96; C. Ralston, *Grass Huts and Warehouses: Pacific Beach Communities of the Nineteenth Century* (Canberra: Australian National University Press, 1977).

16. D. I. Pool, *Te Iwi Maori: A New Zealand Population Past, Present and Projected* (Auckland: University of Auckland Press, 1991).

17. J.-L. Rallu, "Population of the French overseas territories in the Pacific, past, present and projected," *Journal of Pacific History* 26 (1991): 171.

18. For example, C. Macpherson and L. Macpherson, *Samoan Medical Belief and Practice* (Auckland: University of Auckland Press, 1990), pp. 54–58. In a review of McArthur's book, *Island Populations of the Pacific*, Pirie suggested that both early explorers and preliminary archaeological investigations indicate that the population of Samoa at the time of first contact in the late 18th century may have been substantially greater than the estimates from the 1830s, indicating a dramatic collapse, presumably as a result of introduced epidemics. See P. Pirie, "Review of N. McArthur, *Island Populations of the Pacific*," *Australian Geographical Studies* 6 (1968): 175–81. The recent publication by

Macpherson and Macpherson cited at the beginning of this note does not provide any evidence for a massive collapse, though there may have been stagnation or small declines.

19. J.-L. Rallu, *Les Populations océaniennes au xixe et xxe siècles* (Paris: Institut National d'Etudes Demographiques, 1990), pp. 48–49.

20. C. Newbury, *Tahiti Nui: Change and Survival in French Polynesia 1767–1945* (Honolulu: University of Hawaii Press, 1980), pp. 10–11.

21. D. Denoon, *Settler Capitalism* (Oxford: Oxford University Press, 1983).

22. Ibid., pp. 221–24.

23. Ibid., p. 222.

24. Ibid., p. 223.

25. Ibid.

26. Ibid., p. 224.

27. Ibid., p. 217.

28. Macpherson and Macpherson, *Samoan Medical Belief and Practice,* pp. 54–58.

29. P. Pirie, "Population growth in the Pacific islands: The example of Western Samoa," in R. G. Ward, ed., *Man in the Pacific Islands* (Oxford: Oxford University Press, 1972), pp. 198–99.

30. Pool, *Te Iwi Maori,* pp. 88–100. See also M. P. K. Sorrenson, "Land purchase methods and the effect on Maori population, 1865–1901," *Journal of the Polynesian Society* 65 (1956): 183–99.

31. A. W. Crosby, "Hawaiian depopulation as a model for the Amerindian experience," in T. Ranger and P. Slack, eds., *Epidemics and Ideas: Essays on the Historical Perception of Pestilence* (Cambridge: Cambridge University Press, 1992), pp. 175–202; D. E. Stannard, "Recounting the fables of savagery: Native infanticide and the functions of political myth," *Journal of American Studies* 25 (1991): 381–418; Pool, *Te Iwi Maori,* pp. 47–49.

32. Pool, *Te Iwi Maori,* pp. 48–50. These rates are roughly comparable to those reported from the Marquesas cited in Chapter 1.

33. Pool, *Te Iwi Maori,* pp. 75, 79–80.

34. D. E. Stannard, "Disease and infertility: A new look at the demographic collapse of native populations in the wake of Western contact," *Journal of American Studies* 24 (1990): 325–50. See also D. E. Stannard, "The consequences of contact: Toward an interdisciplinary theory of native responses to biological and cultural invasion," in D. H. Thomas, ed., *Columbian Consequences,* vol. 3 (Washington, DC: Smithsonian Institution Press, 1991), pp. 519–89.

35. The Hawaiian figure, based on the ratio of all people aged 0 to 18 to women 18 and above was 83 percent. The Maori ratio a few years earlier was about 70 to 75 percent, using the age groups 0 to 14 and 15 and above. The Hawaiian data are in Schmitt, *Demographic Statistics of Hawaii,* p. 43. The Maori figures are in Pool, *Te Iwi Maori,* p. 72.

36. Pirie, "Population growth"; Pool, *Te Iwi Maori,* pp. 79–80.

37. D. Scarr, *The History of the Pacific Islands: Kingdoms of the Reef* (South Melbourne: Macmillan Company of Australia, 1990), p. 219.

38. R. Crocumbe, ed., *Land Tenure in the Pacific,* rev. ed. (Suva: University of the South Pacific Press, 1987), p. 20.

39. Scarr, *History of the Pacific Islands,* p. 264.

40. M. Meleisea, *The Making of Modern Samoa: Traditional Authority and Colonial Administration in the Modern History of Western Samoa* (Suva: University of the South Pacific Press, 1987), p. 79; Newbury, *Tahiti Nui,* p. 112.

41. S. M. Lambert, *A Yankee Doctor in Paradise* (Boston: Little, Brown, 1941).

42. Pool, *The Maori Population of New Zealand*, pp. 110, 144.

43. F. M. Keesing, *The South Seas in the Modern World* (New York: John Day, 1945), pp. 221–22.

44. P. Schoeffel, "Dilemmas of modernization in primary health care in Western Samoa," *Social Science and Medicine* 19 (1984): 209–16.

45. Meleisea, *The Making of Modern Samoa*, p. 121.

46. Keesing, *The South Seas*, p. 219.

47. Ibid., p. 221.

48. Rallu, *Les Populations océaniennes*, p. 176.

49. Ibid., pp. 154–55.

50. Newbury, *Tahiti Nui*, pp. 142, 197.

51. Rallu, *Les Populations océaniennes*, p. 163.

52. J. Cassel, R. Patrick, and D. Jenkins, "Epidemiological analysis of the health implications of culture change: A conceptual model," *Annals of the New York Academy of Science* 84 (1960): 938–49.

53. R. Redfield, *The Little Community: Viewpoints for the Study of the Human Whole* (Chicago: University of Chicago Press, 1955).

54. I. F. Sunia, "American Samoa: Fa'a Amerika?" in R. Crocombe and A. Ali, eds. *Politics in Polynesia* (Suva: University of the South Pacific Press, 1983), pp. 115–31.

55. Meleisea, *The Making of Modern Samoa*, p. 79.

56. M. H. Fitzgerald and A. Howard, "Aspects of social organization in three Samoan communities," *Pacific Studies* 14 (1990): 31–54.

57. Ibid., p. 45.

58. C. McCuddin, "Overview of American Samoa health care system and health status of the population" (Pago Pago: Division of Planning and Development, Department of Health, L. B. J. Tropical Medical Center, 1989); Department of Health, *Annual Report of the Department of Health, 1986* (Apia: Western Samoa Government Printing Office, 1990), pp. 60–61.

59. For descriptions of the Western Samoa health service, see P. Thomas, "Patterns of disease and health practice in Western Samoa, 1835–1985: Implications for policy," Islands/Australia working paper no. 90/7, 1989; H. Lapsley, "The economics of public health in Western Samoa," Islands/Australia working paper no. 90/5, 1990. Both were published by the National Centre for Development Studies, Research School of Pacific Studies, Australian National University, Canberra.

60. A. R. Omran, "The epidemiologic transition: A theory of the epidemiology of population change," *Milbank Memorial Fund Quarterly* 49 (1971): 509–38; P. T. Baker and D. E. Crews, "Mortality patterns and some biological predictors," in P. T. Baker, J. M. Hanna, and S. Baker, eds., *The Changing Samoans: Behavior and Health in Transition* (Oxford: Oxford University Press, 1986), pp. 93–122; D. E. Crews, "Body weight, blood pressure and the risk of total and cardiovascular mortality in an obese population," *Human Biology* 60 (1988): 417–33; D. E. Crews, "Multiple cause of death and the epidemiological transition in American Samoa," *Social Biology* 35 (1988): 198–213; D. E. Crews, "Multivariate prediction of total and cardiovascular mortality in an obese Polynesian population," *American Journal of Public Health* 79 (1989): 982–86; D. E. Crews and J. D. Pearson, "Cornell Medical Index responses and mortality in a Polynesian population," *Social Science and Medicine* 27 (1988): 1433–37.

61. J. M. Hanna, D. L. Pelletier, and V. J. Brown, "The diet and nutrition of contemporary Samoans," in Baker et al., eds., *The Changing Samoans*, p. 296.

62. P. Zimmet, S. Faaiuso, J. Ainuu, S. Whitehouse, B. Milne, and W. De Boer, "The prevalence of diabetes in the rural and urban Polynesian population of Western Samoa," *Diabetes* 30 (1981): 45–51.

63. Crews, "Body weight."

64. J. Cassel, "Hypertension and cardiovascular disease in migrants: A potential source for clues," *International Journal of Epidemiology* 3 (1974): 204–6.

65. S. T. McGarvey and D. E. Schendel, "Blood pressure of Samoans," in Baker et al., eds., *The Changing Samoans*, p. 374.

66. A. Howard, "Samoan coping behavior," in Baker et al., eds., *The Changing Samoans*, p. 395.

67. McGarvey and Schendel, "Blood pressure of Samoans," p. 380.

68. C. R. Janes, *Migration, Social Change, and Health: A Samoan Community in Urban California* (Stanford, CA: Stanford University Press, 1990), pp. 118–23.

69. Ibid., pp. 124–25.

70. Ibid., p. 123.

71. Howard, "Samoan coping behavior."

72. J. A. Hecht, M. Orans, and C. R. Janes, "Social settings of contemporary Samoans," in Baker et al., eds., *The Changing Samoans*, p. 41.

73. Schoeffel, "Dilemmas of modernization," pp. 211–12.

74. J. T. O'Meara, *Samoan Planters: Tradition and Economic Development in Polynesia* (Fort Worth: Holt, Rinehart and Winston, 1990).

75. Ibid., p. 67.

76. Ibid., pp. 184–89.

77. Ibid., p. 162.

78. Ibid., pp. 189–92.

79. C. Macpherson and L. Macpherson, "Towards an explanation of recent trends in suicide in Western Samoa," *Man* (N.S.) 22 (1987): 305–30.

80. Murphy and Taumoepeau also evoked persistent traditionalism on Tonga to explain what they claim is a low prevalence and incidence of several different psychoses. See H. B. M. Murphy and B. M. Taumoepeau, "Traditionalism and mental health in the South Pacific: A re-examination of an old hypothesis," *Psychological Medicine* 10 (1980): 471–82.

81. E. Beaglehole, *Some Modern Hawaiians*, Research Publication no. 19 (Honolulu: University of Hawaii, 1939), p. 44.

82. Ibid., p. 44.

83. A. Howard, *Ain't No Big Thing: Coping Strategies in a Hawaiian-American Community* (Honolulu: University of Hawaii Press, 1974), p. 4.

84. Beaglehole, *Some Modern Hawaiians*, pp. 100–1.

85. There has in fact been a reawakening of Hawaiian self-consciousness and pride during the past generation. Whether it compares in intensity, breadth, and depth with the Maori renaissance referred to by Beaglehole is beyond the purview of this chapter, as well as beyond my competence to assess.

86. Howard, *Ain't No Big Thing*, pp. 27–28.

87. A. W. Lind, *An Island Community* (Chicago: University of Chicago Press, 1938), p. 325.

88. In 1900 the urban population included only Honolulu, but in 1910 and 1920 it included Hilo as well. See U.S. Bureau of the Census, *Fourteenth Census of the United States Taken in the Year 1920*, vol. 3: *Population 1920, Composition and Characteristics of the Population by States* (Washington, DC: U.S. Government Printing Office, 1922).

89. Honolulu County includes the entire island of Oahu, but the city of Honolulu

accounts for most of the population. The counties other than Honolulu began to grow rapidly in the 1970s with the growth of the tourist industry, which since World War II has replaced sugar as a major source of income. Nordyke, *The Peopling of Hawaii*, pp. 102–5.

90. Lind, *An Island Community*, pp. 308–13.

91. Ibid., p. 311.

92. A. W. Lind, "The ghetto and the slum," *Social Forces* 9 (1931): 210. See also his "Some ecological patterns of community disorganization in Honolulu," *American Journal of Sociology* 36 (1930): 206–20.

93. J. R. McCreary, "Population growth and urbanisation," in E. Schwimmer, ed., *The Maori People in the Nineteen-Sixties* (Auckland: Blackwood and Janet Paul, 1968), p. 202. Hawaiians believed the same thing about their situation; see Howard, *Ain't No Big Thing*, pp. 3–4.

94. A. Ngata, "Maori land settlement," in I. L. G. Sutherland, ed., *The Maori People Today: A General Survey* (Christchurch: Whitcombe and Tombs, 1940), pp. 95–154.

95. H. Belshaw, "Economic circumstances," in Sutherland, ed., *The Maori People Today,* pp. 182–228.

96. McCreary, "Population growth and urbanisation," p. 200.

97. E. Pomare and G. de Boer, *Hauora: Maori Standards of Health: A Study of the Years 1970–1984* (Auckland: Medical Research Council of New Zealand, Special Report Series no. 78, 1988), pp. 28–29; D. Pearson, *A Dream Deferred: The Origins of Ethnic Conflict in New Zealand* (Wellington: Allen & Unwin, 1990), p. 111.

98. N. J. Kent, *Hawaii: Islands Under the Influence* (New York: Monthly Review Press, 1983).

99. Pearson, *A Dream Deferred*, p. 112.

100. A. N. Garwood, ed., *Almanac of the 50 States* (Newburyport, MA: Information Publishers, 1986).

101. Derived from Pearson, *A Dream Deferred*, p. 135.

102. U.S. Bureau of the Census, *Asian and Pacific Islander Population in the United States: 1980,* Report PCC80-2-1E. (Washington, DC: U.S. Government Printing Office, 1988).

103. The definition of Hawaiian and Maori has been a troublesome issue for vital statisticians, demographers, and presumably for many Maoris and Hawaiians as well. Until the 1970 census, Hawaiians had been classified as either Hawaiian or part-Hawaiian, depending on their parentage (whether full or part-Hawaiian ancestry). Starting in 1970, the definition was changed to self-definition. The Hawaii Health Survey of the State Health Department continues to use the initial census definition. The difference in the number of Hawaiians is substantial: Far fewer people define themselves as Hawaiian in the census than are defined as Hawaiian in the Health Department Survey. See Nordyke, *The Peopling of Hawaii,* p. 104. The data I have used are based on the Health Department's definition.

The Maoris' life expectancy data are based on the so-called biological criterion of all those people who are at least half Maori (Pomare and de Boer, *Hauora*, pp. 25–26). There is some reason to believe that even this criterion must include a high proportion of people with less than half Maori ancestry. See Pool, *The Maori Population of New Zealand*, p. 46. In 1981 there were 385,224 people who claimed some Maori ancestry, compared with 279,255 who claimed to be half or more Maori in origin.

Thus both the Hawaiian and Maori life expectancies are based on a "biological" measure having to do with parentage rather than on a measure dependent on "self-definition." On the other hand, the degree of Maori ancestry is more restrictive than the degree of Hawaiian ancestry. It is possible that these differences account for some of the differences in life expectancy reported for recent decades. They are less likely to have confounded the patterns in the interwar and immediate postwar years when intermarriage was much less frequent. See, for example, Howard, *Ain't No Big Thing*, pp. 21–22.

104. D. I. Pool, *Population of New Zealand*, vol. 1, Country Monograph Series no. 12 (Bangkok: United Nations Economic and Social Commission for Asia and the Pacific, 1958), p. 234.

105. S. J. Kunitz, "Mortality change in America, 1620–1920," *Human Biology* 56 (1984): 559–82. Selective migration does not seem to explain the difference adequately.

106. Pool, *Population of New Zealand*, p. 234.

107. R. H. Heighton, Jr., "Physical and dental health," in R. Gallimore and A. Howard, eds., *Studies in a Hawaiian Community: Na Makamaka Nanakuli*, Pacific Anthropological Records no. 1 (Honolulu: Bernice P. Bishop Museum, 1968), p. 121. In 1974 the state of Hawaii passed a law providing virtually universal health coverage. State officials assume that all native Hawaiians are covered. The health changes I am discussing here, however, preceded the availability of such protection.

108. I. A. M. Prior, "Health," in Schwimmer, ed., *The Maori People*, p. 283.

109. Pomare and de Boer, *Hauora*, p. 76.

110. E. Pomare, *Maori Standards of Health: A Study of the 20 Year Period 1955–1975* (Auckland: Medical Research Council of New Zealand, Special Report Series, no. 7, 1980), p. 23.

111. Prior, "Health," pp. 283–84; Pomare, *Maori Standards of Health*, pp. 21–24; Pomare and de Boer, *Hauora*, pp. 72–74.

112. M. A. Look, *A Mortality Study of the Hawaiian People*, R&S Report no. 38 (Honolulu: Hawaii State Health Department, 1982).

113. Department of Statistics, *New Zealand Census of Population and Dwellings, 1981*, volume 8, part A: *New Zealand Maori Population and Dwellings* (Wellington: Department of Statistics, 1982), p. 89.

114. U.S. Bureau of the Census, *Asian and Pacific Islander Population*, p. 841.

115. Pomare and de Boer, *Hauora*, p. 150; L. Le Marchand and L. N. Kolonel, "Cancer: Epidemiology and prevention," *Social Process in Hawaii* 32 (1989): 142.

116. Pomare and de Boer, *Hauora*, p. 153; Le Marchand and Kolonel, "Cancer," p. 140.

117. Pomare and de Boer, *Hauora*, pp. 151–52; Le Marchand and Kolonel, "Cancer," p. 142.

118. E. L. Wegner, "Hypertension and heart disease," *Social Process in Hawaii* 32 (1989): 113–33; Pomare, *Maori Standards of Health*, p. 32.

119. Each of these groups seems to engage in more high-risk behaviors than do nonindigenous peoples in the same countries. See, for example, C. S. Chung, E. Tash, J. Raymond, C. Yasunobu, and R. Lew, "Health risk behaviours and ethnicity in Hawaii," *International Journal of Epidemiology* 19 (1990): 1011–18; P. S. Sachdev, "Behavioural factors affecting physical health of the New Zealand Maori," *Social Science and Medicine* 30 (1990); 431–40.

120. U.S. Bureau of the Census, *Detailed Social and Economic Characteristics, American Samoa*, Report PC80-1-C/D 56 (Washington, DC: U.S. Government Printing Office, 1984); U.S. Bureau of the Census, *Asian and Pacific Islander Population*.

121. I. G. Bertram and R. F. Watters, "The MIRAB economy in South Pacific micros-tates," *Pacific Viewpoint* 26 (1985): 497–519; I. G. Bertram and R. F. Watters, "The MIRAB process: Earlier analyses in context," *Pacific Viewpoint* 27 (1986): 47–59. See

also G. Hayes, "Migration, metascience, and development policy in island Polynesia," *The Contemporary Pacific* 3 (1991): 1–58.

122. S. J. Kunitz, *Disease Change and the Role of Medicine: The Navajo Experience* (Berkeley and Los Angeles: University of California Press, 1983).

123. Native Hawaiians Study Commission, *Report on the Culture, Needs and Concerns of Native Hawaiians,* vols. 1 and 2 (Washington, DC: U.S. Department of the Interior, 1983).

124. D. E. Crews, "Mortality, survivorship and longevity in American Samoa 1950 to 1981" (Ph.D. diss., Pennsylvania State University, 1985), pp. 82–83; R. W. Gardner, *Life Tables by Ethnic Group for Hawaii, 1980,* R&S Report no. 47 (Honolulu: Hawaii State Department of Health, 1984); R. W. Gardner, "Ethnic differentials in mortality in Hawaii, 1920–1970," *Hawaii Medical Journal* 39 (1980): 221–26.

125. A. W. Crosby, *Ecological Imperialism: The Biological Expansion of Europe 900–1900* (Cambridge: Cambridge University Press, 1986); W. M. McNeil, *Plagues and Peoples* (Harmondsworth: Penguin Books, 1976). See also H. Dobyns, *Their Number Become Thinned: Native American Population Dynamics in Eastern North America* (Knoxville: University of Tennessee Press, 1983); A. Mooreheard, *The Fatal Impact* (New York: Harper & Row, 1966).

4

Settler Capitalism and the State in Australia

In Chapter 2 I argued that federal–state relationships were important to explaining differences in mortality patterns of indigenous peoples and that the low life expectancy of Aborigines was due to the fact that Aboriginal affairs have historically been the responsibility of the states. In Chapter 3 I argued that settler capitalism was especially important to accounting for the population decline in New Zealand and Hawaii. In this chapter I temporarily abandon the comparative method in order to examine in more detail the two issues raised in the preceding chapters. I shall do this with a case study of the population history and contemporary health of Aborigines in Queensland in Northern Australia (see Figure 4-1).

It is often claimed that Queensland is not adequately representative of Australia. That is no doubt true in many instances but not, I think, in the history of Aboriginal affairs. Differences from other states seem to me matters of degree rather than kind. But in any case, my purpose is to provide a case study to illustrate my points about state control and settler capitalism, not to describe processes that were identical all across Australia. I shall periodize the story as follows: from 1820 to about the turn of the century, from the turn of the century to the late 1960s, and from the late 1960s to the early 1990s. The first period starts in the 1820s with the expansion of white settlers into what was to become Queensland. It ends with the destruction of most of the indigenous societies they found there, with the closing of the frontier, with the passage of legislation to protect and isolate Aborigines from the white contact, and with Federation. The second period is characterized by the development of a heavily centralized state government committed to economic development and very strong control over the lives of Aborigines. It ends with a change in the Australian constitution that gave the commonwealth government considerable influence over Aboriginal affairs. It is also the time when the Country (later National) party first assumed control of the state government without the Liberals, its former coalition partners. The third period is characterized by increasing conflict between the commonwealth and state governments over the management of Aboriginal affairs and by the emergence for the first time of Aboriginal organizations as significant actors in policymaking and the provision of services.

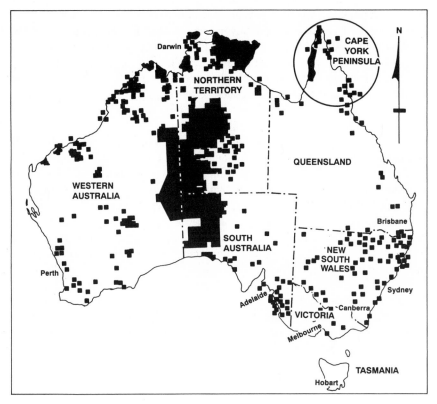

4-1 Map of Australia showing Aboriginal lands and communities, 1985 (Adapted with permission from the author and publisher from J. M. Powell, *An Historical Geography of Modern Australia* [Melbourne: Cambridge University Press, p. 234])

1820–1900

Although Brisbane was first settled in the 1820s, the pastoral frontier really began to expand only in the 1840s. The districts around Brisbane were occupied between 1840 and the early 1860s. Lands to the north and west were occupied in the 1860s.[1] The exception was the Cape York Peninsula, where the rugged terrain combined with Aboriginal resistance to discourage occupation until the discovery of gold in the 1870s.[2] The exception was the Cape York Peninsula, where the rugged terrain combined with Aboriginal resistance to discourage occupation until the discovery of gold in the 1870s.[2]

Aboriginal resistance was substantial wherever pastoralists attempted to establish control over vast tracts. Watering holes were fouled by livestock; vegetation was destroyed; the native flora and fauna on which the Aborigines depended were damaged; and the Aborigines themselves were slaughtered in great numbers whenever resistance was encountered. The most devastating and lethal weapon the settlers possessed was the Native Police, made up of Aborigines from elsewhere who were recruited to hunt, capture, and kill Aborigines who resisted white settlers. Much has been written about the Native Police, a force that was not unique to Queensland.[3] For my purposes what is significant is that the retribution the police exacted from local Aborigines was indiscriminate and massive. Estimates vary and are necessarily imprecise. Raymond Evans wrote that "a reprisal ratio of ten, or even twenty to one in many areas of Northern and Western Queensland cannot be discounted. Indeed, in 1889, Archibald Meston claimed that in the North, as many as fifty Aborigines had been slaughtered to avenge the killing of each European."[4]

In addition to the Native Police, other forms of killing were common. Hunting Aborigines was a sport engaged in by many settlers, who often accompanied the Native Police on raids. Setting out poisoned flour was not uncommon. Starvation resulting from the destruction of the native flora and fauna and epidemics of introduced diseases all were frequent and lethal. The important point is that it was not exotic diseases that were primarily responsible for the devastation of the Aboriginal population in the 19th century, although they contributed mightily. It was, rather, the savagery of the settlers and their calculated slaughter of the indigenous population.

The Native Police were most active and most effective on the pastoral frontier, where guns and horses put them at a great advantage over the lightly armed and unmounted Aborigines. There were, however, other frontiers in Queensland where lethal encounters also occurred: the mining and sea frontiers as well as the rain forest. The Native Police were unable to protect miners as effectively as they had protected pastoralists. Miners traveled alone or in small groups because secrecy was especially important if they were to stake claims to rich finds. They "were often moving into terrain suitable for Aboriginal resistance."[5] And they often moved quickly from one area of exploration to another. Indeed, miners seemed to resort to the use of firearms even "more easily than the pastoralists," for it was ultimately in the pastoralists' interests to reach an accommodation with the Aborigines after they had been pacified, in order to use them as laborers.[6]

On the Cape York Peninsula, where miners, timber-getters, small farmers, and some pastoralists all began to encroach on the Aborigines, conflict was especially prolonged because the rain forest afforded considerable protection. Ultimately the solution was to provide commodities to Aborigines that partially replaced the resources that land acquisition and destruction were denying them. This was an entirely different policy from what had been pursued elsewhere and resulted in the establishment of missions at various places around the Cape York Peninsula, the earliest in the 1870s.[7]

Along the coast of the Cape York Peninsula there was yet a different sort of contact, as seamen in the bêche-de-mer trade used Aborigines as divers and Aboriginal women as sexual objects. These contacts, too, often led to disruption, as men were kidnapped and often never returned and venereal diseases were spread to the population.[8] By 1900 virtually all the Aborigines along the east coast of the Cape York Peninsula were familiar with fishermen. On the west coast the experience differed from north to south. The father south one went, the less contact had there been, and the more dangerous was the travel.[9]

In this context, too, missions were established to protect Aborigines from exploitation. Indeed, they continued to be established well into the 20th century. The consequences were, however, paradoxical. Athol Chase wrote of the north-eastern region of the Cape York Peninsula:

> The coastal plain and ranges were useless for pastoral and agricultural activities, and in any case, they were too remote from lines of communication. Foreigners were interested in sea products and the sparse sandalwood and mineral deposits, so that contact processes appear to have operated in recurrent situations of mutual but temporary cooperation. Aborigines provided the raw labour and local knowledge; foreigners provided the artefacts, food and narcotics that appealed so readily all over Australia. It was a symbiotic relationship and a willing peonage on the part of Aborigines. What the newcomers demanded from the local people was free on their part to give. It did not apparently threaten their lives or their land. Despite population reductions, and new but largely unenforceable laws, these Aborigines were relatively free to pursue their own ends in their own ways.
>
> The major change from foreign intrusion came with the establishment of the Mission.[10]

By the end of the 19th century, then, there were substantial differences in the conditions of the Aborigines in Queensland. Throughout most of the colony the Aboriginal population had been decimated and displaced from their land. Many had been let into the cattle stations, where they found work and were able to remain on or near their own country.[11] Many others clustered for survival on the fringes of towns.[12] On the Cape York Peninsula some people were attracted to missions, and others continued to live a relatively isolated existence on their own lands.

Despite these differences, the perception was widespread that Aborigines were rapidly disappearing. By the 1890s the Aboriginal population of Queensland had been reduced from an estimated 120,000 at the end of the 18th century to perhaps 32,000 (see Table 4-1). That is, over a period of 100 years the population had declined to about 25 percent of its size at the first intensive European contact. Moreover, there was no evidence that the decline would cease. The health of those who survived was being destroyed by venereal diseases, leprosy, an assortment of other infectious diseases, and opium and alcohol use.

It was at this time that the Queensland government's policy began to change in a direction that had been foreshadowed by the missions beginning in the 1870s. Henceforth the policy was to be one of protection and segregation. There were several reasons for the change: among them international pressure[13] and "the increasing political might of the townsmen and their isolation from the harsher conditions of the frontier."[14] Moreover, Aborigines—in the fringe camps especially—were viewed as a source of pollution both moral and physical. White men from the town often sought sexual partners there, thus acquiring as well as introducing venereal diseases. Medical care and treatment were rarely provided. More commonly, the Aborigines were moved to a more distant and less visible location.[15]

The fact that the population was in decline meant that the goal of policy should be to salvage whatever remnants were possible, by means of strict isolation

Table 4–1 Estimated minimum total
Aboriginal and Torres Strait Islander
population of Queensland, 1788–1991

Year	Population
1788	120,000
1861	60,000
1871	50,000
1881	40,000
1891	32,000
1901	27,500
1911	24,500
1921	22,500
1933	22,500
1947	27,500
1954	32,000
1961	37,500
1966	41,500
1971	46,000
1986	61,268
1991	67,012

Sources: For 1788–1971, L. R. Smith, *The Aboriginal Popula-
tion of Australia* (Canberra: Australian National University
Press, 1980), p. 140; for 1986, Australian Bureau of Statistics,
*Census 86—Aboriginal and Torres Strait Islander People in
Queensland* (Canberra: ABS, 1989); for 1991, Aboriginal and
Torres Strait Islander Preliminary Census Counts, unpublished
data provided by the Australian Institute of Health and Welfare,
Canberra, 1993.

(mainly on the Cape York Peninsula) and, if salvage were not possible (and many thought it was not), then "to soothe [*sic*] the pillow of a dying race," as one missionary wrote.[16] In the South where only scattered remnants remained, the goal was to be strict control of the Aborigines' movements, ensuring their availability for work on pastoral stations but otherwise isolating them from white society. Archibald Meston, who carried out a survey of the Aborigines' conditions on behalf of the Queensland government, recommended "absolute exclusion from towns of all but those in rigidly controlled conditions of employment."[17]

This emerging policy was codified in the Aboriginals Protection and Restriction of the Sale of Opium Act, passed by the Queensland legislature in 1897. As the title implies, the act was meant to protect Aborigines by prohibiting the sale of alcohol and opium and by empowering the minister responsible for Aboriginal affairs

through a system of police protectors and reserve superintendents, to control the movements of Aborigines, deny entry to and prevent "escape from" reserves, enter employment contracts on their behalf, hold any funds they may have and control their spending. It allowed for many important administrative matters to be dealt with by Regulations which did not require the consent of Parliament.[18]

Many observers have noted that this act created the framework for the management of Aboriginal affairs in Queensland until well into the 1960s.

1900–1967

The Aboriginals Protection Act was a piece of state legislation. This is important, for it means that in Queensland, as in the other colonies that joined together to become the Commonwealth of Australia in 1901, Aboriginal affairs was firmly a state matter. This continued to be true after federation. Numerous areas of commonwealth–state conflict became evident, but until the late 1960s or early 1970s, Aboriginal affairs was not one of them.

On the other hand, Queensland's policy in regard to the Aborigines was consistent with the so-called White Australia policy that was agreed on at federation. This was a policy aimed at excluding nonwhite immigrants who competed with white workers for jobs and drove down wages. It was not aimed at Aborigines. Nonetheless, Queensland's policy of excluding Aborigines from white communities but allowing them to work in the pastoral industry where it was difficult to hire white workers was consistent with the White Australia policy. This was made explicit by Raphael W. Cilento in 1925; who at the time was director of the Australian Institute of Tropical Medicine, a unit of the Commonwealth Health Department located in Townsville, Queensland. (In the 1930s he became director-general of the Queensland Health Department.) Writing about a survey of the health and living conditions of whites in Queensland, he observed:

> Generally speaking, in no instance did the houses . . . represent the conditions seen in the poorer houses of, say, the poorer towns of Alabama, United States of America, or among the peasants of middle Europe. This is largely due to the fact that Australia has not to contend with the conditions produced in Europe by centuries of vassalage, and that there is practically no aboriginal population in the settled parts of Queensland, and consequently the standard of living among the poorer classes is higher than in the southern States of the United States of America, where approximately one-eighth to one-third of the population of some areas is coloured, and where in the poorer towns white and black are unequal competitors for a hazardous living.[19]

That is, the expulsion of nonwhite immigrants, and the isolation and small numbers of Aborigines, had created the possibility of a white civilization in the tropics. It was the function of tropical medicine and public health to help realize that possibility.

One of the ways in which tropical medicine and public health were to help achieve a white civilization was by making certain that only those Aborigines who were healthy and not carriers of disease were allowed into the wider community. In an unpublished report commissioned by E. M. Hanlon, home secretary of Queensland, and J. W. Bleakley, chief protector of Aborigines, regarding visits to a number of Aboriginal missions and settlements in the early 1930s, Cilento wrote:

I consider that the problem should be treated from the viewpoint of assimilating these native tribes into the population as useful and economic units, particularly in North Queensland. The first basis upon which such a policy might be initiated is the cleaning up of the aboriginals from the point of view of health, and the Palm Islands group is admirably situated to make a clearing station for this purpose.[20]

Later he noted:

The first process—that is, the separation of the medically fit from the unfit—has largely been put into working order. Its steps should be as follows: Transfer through the Palm Islands Settlement of all available aboriginal natives by a deliberate policy of collecting the natives from locality after locality; their distribution through Great Palm to the A.1 grade (white card)—that is to say, young and healthy; the A.2 grade— healthy, but uneducated; and middle aged or over; B.1 grade (yellow card)—young and now healthy, but formerly under treatment for disease; B.2 grade—now healthy, but formerly under treatment for disease, and middle aged or over; C.1 grade (red card)— acutely diseased but curable; C.2 grade—young, chronic, and incurable; C.3 grade— chronic curable, and middle aged or over; or D.1 grade (red card)—mentally infirm, paralysed, or deformed.[21]

These recommendations reflect a broad change in policy at both the national and state levels which was adopted "at a 1937 conference of State and Federal Officials convened by the Federal government," that is, a change from simply protection and preservation to integration.[22] Wearne suggested that this policy, at least in Queensland, was prompted by the recognition that the Aboriginal population had begun to increase since the 1920s: "No longer was there feelings [sic] of shame; sympathy was replaced by paternalism. The debate [in the Queensland legislature] was concerned with making the institution of reserves a success, and preventing the Aboriginal population from disrupting white community standards." Penalties for miscegenation became increasingly harsh, reflecting "a growing concern for the rapidly increasing 'half-caste' population," and the enforcement of segregation became more strict.[23]

It appears that population began to increase both because the reserves did serve a protective function and because in the fringe camp areas there was a good deal of sexual contact between white men and Aboriginal women, resulting in an increase in the "half-caste" population. In regard to the relative effectiveness of the missions and government settlements in protecting the Aborigines, a number of observers commented on the better health of the people living on pastoral stations and missions than of those living on the fringes of white towns and cities.[24] In his unpublished 1932 report, Cilento distinguished between the people living on Palm Island, just off the coast at Townsville, and those living in mainland areas "where the population seen lives subject to minimal restrictions."

The differences are considerable and most important. In the mainland groups, where the aboriginal is merely a hanger-on, or where, though living under native conditions, white settlement has restricted him to some worthless area of ravine or creek bed, only rapidly declining tribal remnants remain, and these are a standing reflection upon the civilisation that permits the conditions producing this situation. In the Settlements, he is commencing to thrive under the care and attention of the Superintendents and the Chief Protector of Aboriginals. Definitely hopeful indications for his future as an individual, and as an economic asset to Australia, are obvious in these localities, and if a rational policy is pursued for a generation, the aboriginal problem can be dealt with in Queensland in a way that will redound to the credit of all Australia. . . .

As stated, the mainland natives are a poor and under-nourished group. During the last few years, owing to the financial stringency, the supplies of food available to them appear to have been minimal—at any rate, the effect of a deficient diet is obvious. This is particularly the case in the southern groups, the situation improving as one goes north into wilder country where foodstuffs and game are more readily accessible, and where the native is less an abject dependent of European families and tenants, or of collections of non-aboriginal colored people.[25]

Regarding miscegenation and the increasing mixed-race population, Cilento went on to observe:

The mainland native resident in relation to the larger towns is considerably worse off and more a menace than any other. It is almost impossible for any aboriginal woman to escape venereal infection in the neighbourhood of (say) Cairns or Innisfail, and among the large foreign and sometimes colored populations that exist in these localities. Promiscuity is encouraged by circumstances almost impossible of governmental control.

An outstanding difficulty is the presence of what may be called the intermediate colored persons—that is to say, those South Sea Island and other mixed races not under the control of the Protector of Aboriginals. These frequently live in morbid surroundings indistinguishable from those of native communities in the Pacific Islands, and invariably centres for infection with hookworm disease, to which is often added venereal disease, and occasionally filariasis and malaria. If, as is stated, these colored persons are outside the jurisdiction of any governmental branch, I am of the opinion that the law should be amended to bring under the direct control of the Chief Protector of Aboriginals any family of colored or partly colored blood living under native conditions, or under circumstances menacing to the community from the point of view of health, or under circumstances in which they are liable to become a charge upon the community.[26]

Thus public health policy reflected the goals of Aboriginal policy more broadly and helped rationalize segregation, even as integration remained the goal. For their own good and that of the white population, strengthening the laws controlling contact between the races was thought justified until the Aborigines were ready to take their place in the larger society. Changes in the 1897 act by the Queensland legislature in 1939 did just that. Indeed, life "under the act" became increasingly oppressive, as the autobiographies recorded by Bill Rosser reveal.[27] Moreover, even though integration was the stated ultimate aim, it was remarkably difficult to be freed from supervision and control, and the freedom could always be revoked for what was thought to be a transgression of community norms. According to the annual reports of the director of the Department of Native Affairs (the successor to the office of Chief Protector of Aboriginals), throughout the 1940s and 1950s only about 100 people a year were released from the supervision of the act.[28]

The policy of assimilation had been adopted in 1937, but it was elaborated more clearly at the federal level in 1951 when the stated goal was that all Aborigines "shall attain the same manner of living as other Australians, enjoying the same rights and privileges, accepting the same responsibilities, observing the same customs, and being influenced by the same beliefs, hopes and loyalties."[29] As we have seen, the reality in Queensland was to enforce segregation and control rather than integration. But that began to change in 1957, at the time when minerals were discovered on Aboriginal lands.[30]

Bauxite had been discovered in 1955 at Weipa, a Presbyterian mission on the west coast of the Cape York Peninsula. When the Country party/Liberal party coalition attained power in Queensland in 1957, it began to pursue a very active policy of economic development that involved attracting international corporations with capital to invest in the extraction of natural resources. Bauxite mining at Weipa was very high on the list of projects. The story of the removal of Aborigines from the mission and the loss of hundreds of thousands of hectares of the reserve to the Commonwealth Aluminum Corporation (Comalco) has been told numerous times and need not detain us here.[31] Likewise, in 1965 similar arrangements were made with Alcan, a Canadian corporation, for 1,373 square kilometers of land that extended into the Mapoon Aboriginal Reserve, also on the west coast of the Cape York Peninsula. In this case a police raid resulted in the residents of the reserve being forcibly rounded up and removed to New Mapoon, at the northern end of the peninsula. In neither case did the Aboriginal communities acquire shares in the companies or a significant number of jobs at the mines. In each case, as well as in a similar episode in the 1970s, the state government rejected the rights of Aborigines to freehold title (including mining rights) to the land on which their reserves were located. In each case, too, the rationale was that the granting of such rights would mean that development would not occur, or if it did, that only Aborigines would benefit and white Queenslanders would be relegated to the status of second-class citizens. Which is to say, a segregated society would be created which, in the altered context of natural resource extraction, was no longer tolerable.

I have said that the policies of the 1930s seem to have been due in part to the recognition that the Aborigines had begun to increase in number and that something had to be done to deal more positively with them. There is scattered evidence that throughout this period Aboriginal health continued to improve. The increase in population from its nadir in the 1920s and 1930s is one indication. Improvements in infant mortality from the 1930s through the 1960s is another, although the data exist only for people living in Aboriginal communities, not in fringe camps or urban areas (see Table 4-2). Moreover, estimates of average annual birth rates and death rates indicate an increase of the former and a decrease of the latter from 1921 to 1936 (see Table 4-3).

These improvements, particularly in the 1950s and 1960s, seem to have been associated with immunization campaigns, which were reported regularly in the annual reports of the director of native affairs in those years, as well as attempts at improving the availability of clean water, adequate housing, and waste disposal facilities. Nonetheless, by the late 1960s the evidence still indicated substan-

Table 4–2 Infant mortality rates, various Queensland Aboriginal populations, 1933–1990

Date	Population	Rate/1,000 live births
1933–35[a]	Taior, Ngentjin, Yir Yiront, Yir Mel (near Edward and Mitchell rivers)	412
1947–72[b]	Kowanyama (Mitchell River)	95
1940–69[b]	Edward River	113
1954–58[c]	Woorabinda	181
1955–57[d]	Doomadgee	297
1957–60[e]	Lockhart	100
1959[f]	Palm Island	70
1953–59[g]	Cherbourg	236
1960–69[g]	Cherbourg	135
1960–69[h]	Edward River	144
1962–66[i]	Cherbourg, Woorabinda, Palm Island, Mitchell River, Edward River, Aurukun, Weipa, Mornington Island, Doomadgee	112
1963–73[j]	Palm Island	41
1970–72[k]	Cherbourg	40
1972–76[l]	12 communities	72
1973–81[m]	14 communities	54.1
1982–90[m]	14 communities	21.6

[a] R. L. Sharp, "An Australian Aboriginal population," *Human Biology* 5 (1940):481–507.

[b] J. C. Taylor, "Aboriginal child health: Anthropologist's report," *30th Annual Report,* Queensland Institute of Medical Research (Brisbane: Government Printer, 1975), p. 23.

[c] Queensland Department of Native Affairs, *Annual Reports of the Director* (Brisbane: Government Printer, 1954–58).

[d] Queensland Department of Native Affairs, *Annual Reports of the Director* (Brisbane: Government Printer, 1955–57).

[e] Queensland Department of Native Affairs, *Annual Reports of the Director* (Brisbane: Government Printer, 1957, 1959, 1960 [no data for 1958]).

[f] Queensland Department of Native Affairs, *Annual Reports of the Director* (Brisbane: Government Printer, 1959).

[g] A. E. Dugdale, "Infant feeding, growth and mortality: A 20-year study of an Australian Aboriginal community," *Medical Journal of Australia* 2 (1980):382.

[h] J. C. Taylor, "A pre-contact Aboriginal medical system on Cape York Peninsula," *Journal of Human Evolution* 6 (1977):419–32.

[i] D. G. Jose, M. H. R. Self, and N. D. Stallman, "A survey of children and adolescents on Queensland Aboriginal settlements, 1967," *Australian Paediatric Journal* 5 (1969):71–88.

[j] W. J. Fysh, R. Davison, D. Chandler, and A. E. Dugdale, "The weights of Aboriginal infants: A comparison over 20 years," *Medical Journal of Australia,* special supplement, June 4, 1977, pp. 13–15.

[k] A. E. Dugdale, "Infant feeding, growth and mortality: A 20-year study of an Australian Aboriginal community," *Medical Journal of Australia* 2 (1980):382.

[l] J. W. Cox, "Infant mortality in 12 Aboriginal settlements: Queensland, 1972–76," *Medical Journal of Australia,* Special Supplement, February 24, 1979, pp. 8–9.

[m] R. Hogg and N. Thomson, "Fertility and mortality of Aborigines living in the Queensland aboriginal communities, 1972–1990," Aboriginal and Torres Strait Islander Health Series no. 8 (Canberra: Australian Institute of Health and Welfare, 1992).

Table 4–3   Estimates of vital rates per 1,000 for total Aboriginal population of
Queensland, 1921–36

Five years centered on	Average birthrate	Average deathrate	Average rate of increase
1921	16.7	21.5	−4.8
1926	18.1	17.8	+1.2
1931	20.6	19.4	+1.2
1936	24.4	18.2	+6.2

Source: L. R. Smith, *The Aboriginal Population of Australia* (Canberra: Australian National University Press,
1980), p. 139.

tial health problems. The data are sparse but suggest there was little improvement
in the growth of children from the early 1950s to the early 1970s. At Cherbourg
in 1953, median weight at 12 months was 8.25 kg for boys and 7.84 for girls; in
1963, 8.25 and 8.01; and in 1972, 8.22 and 8.44 for boys and girls, respectively.
Median weights for boys and girls on Palm Island were 8.35 and 7.5 in 1963 and
8.68 and 7.24 in 1973.[32] Virtually all these measurements were at the 10th
percentile of the Harvard standards.

Similarly, two surveys of a larger number of communities in the late 1960s
indicated that in general, high proportions of children were below the 10th
percentile of weight for age.[33] In four communities the proportions ranged between 39 and 56 percent; and in two others they were 18 and 16 percent. In a
discussion of these two surveys, Jose and Welch observed:

> Four periods of growth were evident: a period of early normal growth (birth to six
> months), a period of complete or partial cessation of growth (six months to two years), a
> period of slow "catch up" (two to six years), and a period of rapid "catch up" (seven to
> 11 years).[34]

They also remarked that "slowing or cessation of growth in Aboriginal children
aged between six months and three years has been observed in many areas of
Australia."[35] Thus although there was evidence of real improvements in health
up to and including the 1960s, there was also plentiful evidence that malnutrition
and other health problems of infancy and childhood persisted at levels much
above those observed in the non-Aboriginal Australian population.

The end of this period saw two developments of profound significance. The
first was the referendum in 1967 that changed "two clauses in the Federal
Constitution discriminating against Aborigines: section 127, which excluded
Aborigines of the full descent from national census counts and section 51
(XXVI), which prohibited the Federal government from passing laws relating to
Aborigines living in the Australian States."[36] The second development was the
ascent to the premiership of Queensland by Joh Bjelke-Petersen in 1968.

The passage of the referendum was by an overwhelming majority, about 90
percent of people voting in favor of the changes. On the other hand, there were

mainly rural electorates where Aborigines were highly visible, and where substantial proportions voted against the referendum.[37] The greatest rates of approval were in the urban eastern electorates. These patterns support the point made in Chapter 2 that urbanites have been more likely to support rights of indigenous people because indigenous people are simply not a salient part of their everyday existence and do not compete for resources.

The referendum gave the commonwealth government the right to pass laws regarding Aborigines. It did not deny the states their preexisting rights to do the same. That is, the new power was concurrent rather than exclusive, which created new sources of conflict between the commonwealth and state governments and resulted in fewer advances for the Aborigines than the advocates of the referendum had expected.[38] In Queensland under Premier Bjelke-Petersen, the conflict was particularly acrimonious.

1967–1989

The context within which health services for Aborigines evolved through the 1970s and 1980s in Queensland was conflict between the federal and state governments over policies of self-determination on the one hand and assimilation on the other.[39] Self-determination, later called self-management, was the federal policy adopted after the 1967 referendum.

> Self-determination is essentially an international principle which grew out of the effect of foreign occupation on the peoples of certain territories. In the Australian context it was a seemingly useful policy title with principles which could, in a governmental sense, erode the political residue of assimilation and the policies that went before. The modern concept of self-determination developed out of world wars. It was supposed that, with supervision from the League of Nations, territories under allied occupation would eventually progress along the path of self-determination. Following World War II, the United Nations Charter (article 73) recognized that self-determination was a principle supporting "the interests of the inhabitants of . . . territories." The idea was that the political aspirations of people would be acknowledged within the international context of sovereignty.[40]

Assimilation continued to be the policy that Queensland followed, however. It meant, in essence, that Aborigines would become part of the larger Australian public, without special rights that were the result of their membership in a particular racial group or corporate community such as an Aboriginal reserve.

The practical consequences of these differences in regard to land rights and control over natural resources were, as we have seen, profound. Perhaps best known and most thoroughly documented were the disputes among the two levels of government and Aboriginal peoples themselves over the status of the Presbyterian missions at Mornington Island and Aurukun, the former in the Gulf of Carpenteria and the latter on the northwest coast of the Cape York Peninsula. The story has been told elsewhere.[41] Suffice it to say here that in each case the Aboriginal communities wanted to continue their relationship with the Presbyterian church (which by that time had become part of the Uniting church), in opposition to the state's announced intention of assuming management of the reserves (on March 31, 1978). Federal legislation was hurriedly passed to give Aborigines the right to manage their own communities, but before the act could be passed, the state de-gazetted the reserves, meaning that their legal status was changed from being reserves to being local shires, or counties. As shires, the federal legislation was not applicable, and the state retained control over the natural resources which, in the case of Aurukun, were considerable.

These same issues of local community control (or self-determination) and assimilation ran through debates and discussions of the provision of services after the federal government began to fund health programs for Aborigines in the early 1970s. Indeed, these larger conflicts over land rights and control of resources made the debates over health services even more acrimonious.

In the early 1970s when the federal government began to support health programs for Aborigines, studies by the Queensland Institute of Medical Research had recently been published.[42] These drew attention to the continuing high rates of infant mortality, malnutrition, and infectious diseases among the children of a number of the major reserves on the Cape York Peninsula. Indeed, the association between malnutrition and diarrhea in infants and children was a major subject of research in the international health field in the late 1960s; increasing attention was being paid to it by the World Health Organization; and it was embarrassing to discover conditions among indigenous peoples in Western liberal democracies that were similar to those found in the so-called Third World.[43] Thus when federal support became available to state governments for health programs, infant mortality and acute malnutrition became the major targets.

In Queensland the major surveys had been done on the larger Aboriginal communities, but subsequent observations suggested that the problem was more widespread in the Aboriginal population and occurred as well in town reserves and in fringe camps located on the edges of towns and cities. For instance, in a survey done in 1970 by D. I. A. Musgrave, soon to become the founding director of the Aboriginal Health Program of the Queensland Health Department, he observed:

> Evidence of malnutrition is apparent in every centre where Aborigines exist, whether on Communities or in Reserves or in fringe areas of the townships. Recent researches by Drs. Jose, Galbraith and Stuart provide evidence of this in twelve Communities. Personal observation tends to indicate that their findings are fairly general throughout the whole Aboriginal Community. Malnutrition is perhaps the most prevalent underlying disease process in Aboriginal children.[44]

Musgrave went on to describe the inadequate diets and housing and the general living conditions of the Aborigines in the various communities he visited. The exceptions were people living in newly built homes in towns, who he thought displayed great pride and were caring for themselves and their children at a higher standard. He believed that not only were wages too low, often providing an incentive for people to remain unemployed and collect social welfare payments, but that also what money was available was spent unwisely because of the Aborigines' lack of adequate education as well as their gambling and excessive use of alcohol. According to Musgrave, "there are numerous cases of abuse of money by Aborigines in which the family is allotted only a very small amount of the budget to buy food, sometimes as little as $4.00 per week. Associated with this are frequently problems of gambling and excessive indulgence in alcohol."[45]

In urban areas there also was evidence of serious health problems. For example, a study of weight for age (a measure of chronic malnutrition) in Aboriginal youngsters served by an Aboriginal medical service in Brisbane in the mid-1970s indicated that between 31 and 47 percent (depending on age) were below the 5th percentile of the international standard in use at the time. The lowest proportion (33 percent) was found among the children of married women; the highest (49 percent) among "supporting mothers" (single mothers).[46] Because these were children examined in a medical practice, they may have been a biased sample of the urban Aboriginal population. Nonetheless, the results indicated that the nutritional status in urban areas was not good.

Eckermann's study in the early 1970s of a small Aboriginal population in a place she called Rural Town in southwest Queensland indicated that about half of the adults drank to excess. She traced this to two "vicious circles": cultural exclusion, which helped further the process of social disintegration, and a socioeconomic environment "distinguished by few financial resources and unskilled or semi-skilled employment within an ever growing atmosphere of chronic poverty."[47] This was partially the result of the restructuring of primary industries, which further restricted economic possibilities. The problem was not lack of knowledge of the white society and its ways, but poverty and prejudice.[48] For example, Eckermann tells of the difficulties of obtaining health care in the town even when it was "free."[49] Thus in both a small rural town and in the major city in the state, poverty and its attendant health risks and problems of access to services continued to be pervasive.

When the State Health Department's Aboriginal Health Program was established in 1972, children were screened to assess their growth patterns. The children were selected from a large number of communities (the Queensland term for the major missions and government-run settlements), reserves (small settlements on government land near towns), fringe settlements (squatters on land near the edges of towns), and towns. Wasting was the characteristic of most concern. This is defined as low weight for height and is thought to reflect acute malnutrition rather than the chronic malnutrition reflected in low weight for age. "Based on present evidence, some wasting is considered to exist when weight is less than 90% of standard weight for length."[50] The results of the first screenings in each population showed that the unweighted average of the proportion of wasted children was 38 percent (a range of 29 to 68 percent) in the major communities and 22.2 percent (0 to 43 percent) in all the other populations. Thus, although in general the children in the communities experienced the highest prevalence of acute malnutrition, there was much overlap with other Aboriginal children in Queensland.

It was clear from his 1970 report that Musgrave saw Aboriginal health problems in a broad context, one consistent with the views prevailing in Queensland and elsewhere at the time, though increasingly being contested.

> This hunter–gatherer nomadic society has now been nearly destroyed and Aborigines are required to live virtually in the one place in structured dwellings and to eat unfamiliar foodstuffs which must first be purchased and not hunted for and which fact, in turn, demands the pursuit of occupations entirely foreign to the traditional ways of passing the day. It is not hard to understand the resistance to change of this sort.[51]

He went on to say that the consequence of these changes was that houses were not cared for properly nor was money spent wisely.

> There is a distinct relationship, therefore, between this cultural problem and the problems of health and nutrition. All of these problems become less as the Aborigine becomes better educated and better employed and situated more in the midst of the European community. These problems are minimal in those families which have been adequately housed in provincial towns and who have adequate employment on at least Award wages.[52]

For all these reasons Musgrave recommended not only higher wages but also the destruction of fringe camps and the removal of people to adequate housing in European towns, as well as the expatriation of children, not later than their 12th birthday, to boarding schools and foster homes away from the "demoralising and stultifying atmosphere of the Communities." "While they continue to lack sufficient education to be able to think their own problems through clearly, one can expect the continuance of such problems as gambling and alcoholism."[53] He concluded that his various observations indicated "the need for the eventual relocation of all community dwellers and all sub-standard fringe dwellers into good housing in towns, into good occupations and with their children attending good schools, and that the concept of the 'Assisted Aborigine' eventually be abandoned for the sake of his dignity and morale."[54]

Thus the poor health of Aborigines was the result of their poverty, marginalization, and lack of education and employment opportunities. This was a diagnosis with which virtually no one would have taken exception, then or now. The prescription for change was more contentious, however, for by 1970 assimilation into the larger society was no longer universally accepted as the best solution to the problem of Aboriginal disadvantage. But it continued to be the dominant belief in Queensland, and Musgrave saw it as a task that required far more than health services. It was, rather, a task in which a variety of state agencies needed to cooperate. Instead of the fragmentation that he and others agreed characterized the services provided by a plethora of often competing state agencies, he argued that there needed to be an integrated approach.[55] The role of the federally funded Aboriginal Health Program was to focus primarily on infant and child health.

The federal government did not support only one health program in Queensland or anywhere else. In addition to providing money to state health departments, support was also given to nonstate agencies, often community-based Aboriginal Medical Services as well as other agencies. This soon became a most contentious issue.

The federal government's health policy as enunciated by R. I. Viner, the minister for Aboriginal affairs in the coalition Liberal party/National party government of Prime Minister Malcolm Fraser, was based on the concept of self-management (the National party/Liberal party modification of self-determination[56]), which underlay Aboriginal policy more generally.

In the Aboriginal health field, this is reflected in the focus on the individual community in health service provision, with the community increasingly identifying its health needs and determining priorities for resource allocation. Emphasis is placed on utilisation of the community's traditional health resources, and on adaptation of Western medical practices in response to cultural differences, as when, for example, traditional healers work alongside salaried doctors, nurses and Aboriginal health-workers. Particular emphasis is placed on the development of Aboriginal control and management skills.[57]

Viner went on: "My directive requires the Department of Aboriginal Affairs to place the community and its people at the centre of any aspect of community development, and sees Aboriginal commitment to and involvement in identifying health needs and all aspects of planning, management and delivery of services as essential to any real progress."[58]

This policy created much distress in the state-administered Aboriginal Health Program, for several reasons. First, other programs were seen to be competing for a limited supply of money. Second, these other programs were viewed as nonprofessional and often as pursuing a political agenda. And third, Queensland had a long history of political centralization, for example, in the management of its hospital system, which was the only free statewide system in Australia until the development of national health insurance.[59] The sort of decentralization that was being encouraged by federal policy was clearly a threat to this established bureaucratic and political culture. In 1978, at hearings in Brisbane held by the federal government's House of Representatives Standing Committee on Aboriginal Affairs, as well as in documents published by the Department of Health of Queensland, Musgrave took strong exception to the policies being pursued.

The writer is aware that the Commonwealth Department of Aboriginal Affairs pursued its own investigations into the demography and health needs of Aborigines in Queensland. The intention was to determine where the allocations for future funding should be directed. There is a risk that significant funding will be directed to projects which can only be considered as ad hoc and inexpert, and made by grant, and that this will be matched by an equivalent reduction in the level of funding to State Government Agencies concerned with provision of health services for Aborigines especially the Aboriginal Health Programme which is of proven effectiveness already and which deserves expansion rather than curtailment. This is a highly undesirable trend because of a number of reasons:

(a) The Ministerial guidelines have been drafted without regard to planning by the State Health Department. Expertise of State Government Departments is being ignored and will be lacking in the conduct of these new services.

(b) With the increasing development of various community health services operated by the State Government, there will be duplication of those services where aboriginal patients are concerned.

(c) This trend must lead to further separation of the aboriginal population or part of it from the community at large and will be detrimental to the integration of Aborigines into the whole community.

(d) Health of Aborigines must suffer as a result of the limitations incumbent in such ad hoc services.

(e) The fact that "special" services appear to be provided for Aborigines alone and not to other minority groups, can be expected to antagonise the rest of the community, more or less, depending upon locality. The existence of an unhealthy aboriginal population, served by a separate inadequate health service, should also be considered in the context of other initiatives relating to the advancement of Aborigines but which are tending to set them apart from the rest of the population.

(f) By coming to depend upon inexpert and ad hoc services, the health of Aborigines is less likely to improve than if services were to be provided through a co-ordinated system wherein the rights and responsibilities of State Government Departments were preserved.

(g) The longer a significant proportion of Aborigines suffer from health problems at a greater level than the rest of the community, the greater will be the expenditure required to attempt to overcome these health problems and also that required to provide for various related unemployment benefit and social welfare payments arising out of illness. At the same time, Aborigines who are ill or disadvantaged through alcoholism or mental health problems which might have been corrected, will be precluded from seeking employment and will suffer accordingly, as will their families.[60]

The House of Representatives hearings coincided with the conflict over the status of the former missions at Mornington Island and Aurukun. The reference to a survey sponsored by the Department of Aboriginal Affairs seems to be a study made jointly by the Aborigines and Torres Strait Islanders Legal Service and the Foundation for Aboriginal and Islander Research Action and funded by the federal government. It formed the basis for a submission to a Queensland state commission whose function was to advise the state's minister for Aboriginal and Islanders advancement and fisheries on policies regarding Aboriginal and Islander affairs in the state. The survey of 912 Aboriginal and Islander adults living on reserves and 879 living in towns found that the vast majority living on reserves wanted the commonwealth (federal) government to replace the state government as the body responsible for making laws; wanted Aboriginal and Islander ownership of reserves; and wanted community councils on each reserve to control decision making on a large number of matters, including housing, mining, business enterprises, and the availability of liquor. The opinions of people living in towns were similar.[61] Clearly, this survey represented a repudiation of the state government's control of Aboriginal and Islander affairs in favor of federal support for community control. Like Musgrave, the state commission to which the survey was submitted was dismissive:

> The Commonwealth Government, through an unrealistic degree of idealism, appears to be committed to a dangerous policy of separate development. . . . Presently the Commonwealth Government appears to be enthusiastically accepting that total possession and use of traditional tribal land areas will restore racial pride, produce economic comfort, reduce delinquency and cure alcoholism.
>
> Commissioners honestly and seriously question this approach and feel that the best programme for Aboriginal and Islander development lies in eventual integration into the broader structure of society.[62]

Further complicating the scene was the fact that in April 1979, Prime Minister Malcolm Fraser had written to the state premiers to say that

> the Commonwealth considers that the inclusion of the States' Aboriginal populations in general revenue reimbursement calculations makes it appropriate for the States to provide in their own general programs at least a pro rata share for Aboriginals. This means that any additional or special services for Aboriginals should not be either the exclusive responsibility of the Commonwealth, or be seen indefinitely as matters falling outside normal State Government service delivery.[63]

This clearly meant that many services were expected to be taken over by the states. And indeed that is what happened, for even though the current dollar amount allocated to the Aboriginal Health Program remained stable, there was a decline in real terms of about 30 percent from 1983/84 financial year to the 1990/91 financial year.[64] In memos from high-ranking members of the State Health Department there was agreement that the state should assume responsibility as the commonwealth withdrew, which occurred on June 30, 1992.

It is not necessary to describe in any detail the debates during the 1980s. The issues were essentially the same as in the 1970s: community-based programs supported by the commonwealth in competition with state government programs also supported, but at diminishing levels, by the commonwealth. The concerns of the state officials continued to be the same as well: the use of health programs run by nonprofessionals without "expertise" to advance political agendas inimical to the interests of all Queenslanders. For example, the notes of a meeting of officers from the State Departments of Health and of Aboriginal and Islander Advancement in 1981 concluded:

> In the essential competition for Federal funding which exists between the private health organisations and the State, an important but fallacious argument is repeatedly offered, not only by the private organisations themselves but also by the Commonwealth authorities. This argument is predicated upon the premise that self-determination by Aborigines requires that they should plan and control their own health services. Except in some of the policy aspects, this is false. Whereas Aboriginal participation is good and desirable up to the level at which it is effective, in the context of service delivery, self-determination by Aborigines is a separate issue, a political issue. It is an issue which is

related to policy rather than practice and it does not depend upon the proportion of Aborigines participating in any particular service designed for their benefit or welfare. Of course, for the private organisations or Federal authorities to acknowledge this, would be to expose the ploy wherein they are using the promotion of private Aboriginal health services as a tactic to advance the objective of Aboriginal self-determination rather than the objective of health improvement of Aborigines.[65]

There are two points to be made here. First, it was clear that the state officials viewed the competing Aboriginal medical services as nothing more than a vehicle for self-determination, whereas they chose to view their own stance as apolitical and concerned only with the disinterested provision of expertly and professionally guided services. Moreover, they seem to have viewed the alliance between the commonwealth government and the Aboriginal medical services as a comfortable one, which was very far from being the case. There was, rather, mutual suspicion, based on the perception of the Aboriginal medical services that commonwealth bureaucrats were excessively controlling and holding them to standards that no health care providers could be reasonably expected to meet.[66] On the commonwealth's side there was undoubtedly anxiety that money was being spent irresponsibly and for purposes that were not, strictly speaking, medical.

Second, the debates reflect the reality of the continuing fragmentation of services, which had been noted as early as 1970 in Musgrave's original report. Arguably, this fragmentation had even been exacerbated by the entry of the commonwealth government into the fray. The commonwealth government seemed to want to guide Aboriginal health policy while at the same time expecting the state governments to continue to provide services. No wonder that Musgrave wrote in exasperation in 1978: "If the intention is to withdraw, then the Commonwealth Department of Aboriginal Affairs should also refrain now from attempting to determine without consultation with State Health Authorities how health services for Aborigines should be developed. Without the money, the advice is not wanted."[67]

In 1991, more than 20 years after the commonwealth government's entry into Aboriginal health affairs, the Human Rights and Equal Opportunity Commission concluded on the basis of hearings on the Cape York Peninsula:

> As a result of the fragmentation of responsibility for the provision of health services the Aboriginal and Torres Strait Islander residents of Cooktown, Wujal Wujal and Hopevale are confronted with gaps in some areas of service delivery (as graphically illustrated by the lack of ambulance facilities) and duplication in other areas. A disjointed approach to planning, delivery and evaluation of health services has led to ad hoc coverage and quality of service, retarding the impact on overall health improvement.[68]

Among the most obviously deficient programs were those for the prevention and treatment of alcohol and substance abuse, as well as mental health services. In his testimony before the House of Representatives Standing Committee on Aboriginal Affairs in 1978, Musgrave had stated that the original "targets of the campaign [of the Aboriginal Health Program] would be the elimination of malnutrition and infectious disorders of children and, once established, the harder task of elimination of the problems affecting adults, particularly alcohol abuse, venereal diseases, and so on."[69] But little was ever done in this regard, although beginning in the 1980s, annual reports from the Department of Health increasingly acknowledged the severity of adult health problems and the need for intervention.

That adult health was an overwhelming concern of Aborigines was revealed in a survey of the opinions of Aborigines and Torres Strait Islanders in the Townsville region in 1991. The results indicated that the most significant health problems were thought to be alcohol and drug abuse and domestic violence.[70] It is thus significant that a survey of mental health services for Aborigines in 1991, appropriately subtitled "Fragmented and Forgotten," concluded that at least 60 percent of residents of many Aboriginal communities were in some need of mental health assistance but that such services were nonexistent. The authors went on to say that the de facto health policy of the state was based on the highly problematic assumption that " 'equal access' means delivering services which are identical to each consumer, and a conviction that the differing health values and interpretations of non-English background consumers are of no consequence to the health care or medical practitioner."[71]

Indeed, a remarkably candid analysis of health services for Queensland Aborigines and Islanders by the director of the Aboriginal Health Program in 1990 concluded that there had been "difficulties in co-operation" between state agencies and Aboriginal medical services: "There is still considerable mistrust (in both directions)"; "there is insufficient co-ordination."[72] As to problems of substance abuse, he noted that the State Health Department's Division of Alcohol and Drug Dependence Services had provided only "four dedicated staff to target a population of 61,268 Aboriginal and Torres Strait Islander people in Queensland;" many of the counselors trained by the division were unemployed; and those who were employed got very limited assistance from the division.[73] He concluded:

Overall Aboriginal Health policy has not been adequately co-ordinated in Queensland because:

- From the Health Department perspective there has been no single point of accountability for development of policy and guidelines for both curative and preventive services.
- Curative services are developed by Public Hospitals Branch, Nursing Services and Health and Medical Services.
- Some curative services have until recently been under the control of another department (Department of Family Services and Aboriginal and Islander Affairs)
- Preventive services in the Aboriginal Health Programme have been responsible to the Assistant Director General (Community) and hence to the Department Executive. . . .

From the Aboriginal and Torres Strait Islander community perspective the Aboriginal and Islander Health Advisory Council (AIHAC), has worked tirelessly and raised many important issues but

- the Aboriginal and Torres Strait Islander Community has not recognized AIHAC as being truly representative of the Aboriginal and Torres Strait Islander community.
- the AIHAC has not been adequately resourced.
- the AIHAC has often not been consulted or informed when important policy decisions in Aboriginal and Torres Strait Islander health have been made.[74]

What, then, were the consequences of these policy battles for the health of Aborigines? Sadly, Queensland's policy of assimilation has meant that race is not listed on birth or death certificates. Thus virtually the only data available come from the Aboriginal Health Program itself, which kept scrupulously careful records of vital events and infant and child development from its inception in 1972 to 1990, but only for the 14 major Communities where the bulk of its services were provided and where the populations were most completely enumerated. In regard to infant mortality, as Table 4-2 indicates, the evidence is unequivocal: Rates continued to decline dramatically over the 18-year period.

Other measures, however, showed little or no change. For example, Hogg and Thomson observed that "from 1972 to 1990, the proportion of babies of low birthweight born to Aboriginal women living in the communities (less than 2,500 grams) has remained between 14 and 16 percent."[75] This is about three times the rate among non-Aborigines in Queensland.[76]

Moreover, studies of growth and development indicate little change in chronic malnutrition as measured by weight for age.[77] Recall that I said earlier that there had been little change from the 1950s to the 1960s and that the mean and median weights for age had often been found to be around the 10th percentile of the Harvard standards. A study comparing growth patterns of infants at a mission in the Gulf of Carpentaria from 1966–72 to 1973–76 showed that among boys, the mean weight at a year of age had increased from 9.28 to 9.52 kg, or from just below the 20th percentile to just below the 30th.[78] In Mount Isa in 1973–76, Aboriginal boys weighed 9.49 kg at a year of age. On the other hand, among girls on the mission there was no improvement: They averaged 8.74 kg in the first period and 8.63 in the second (below the 30th percentile). In Mount Isa the Aboriginal girls at a year of age averaged 8.68 kg in 1973–76. The pattern of faltering growth described by Jose and Welch could be detected in both periods. Likewise, a study of growth of children from five Queensland Aboriginal communities in the 1970s showed the same pattern.[79] At 1 year of age the boys weighed on average 9.1 kg (about the 15th percentile), and the girls, 8.6 kg (about the 20th percentile).

There is scattered evidence, then, that from the late 1960s to the early 1970s there may have been an increase in weight at 1 year of age from below the 10th to around the 20th percentile or even a little more, depending on the communities in which the measurements were made. Before that time, however, the little evidence available indicates essentially no change. The pattern of faltering growth persisted into the 1970s even as weight at 1 year of age seemed to increase slightly.

From the early 1970s onward, data have become more generally available since the Aboriginal Health Program has been very concerned to monitor growth accurately. Figures 4-2 and 4-3 display the results of the screenings, comparing

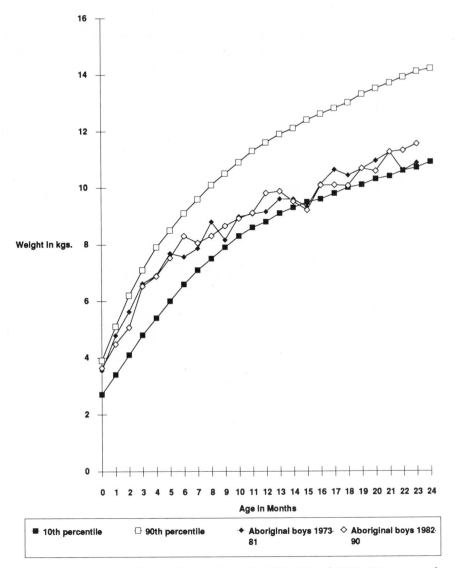

Figure 4-2 Mean weights of Aboriginal boys in 1973–81 and 1982–90, compared with Harvard standards. (*Source:* S. J. Kunitz, R. Streatfield, G. Santow, and A. de Craen, "The health of populations on North Queensland Aboriginal communities: Change and continuity," *Human Biology*, vol. 66, no. 5, 1994. Reprinted with permission of Wayne State University Press.

mean weights (in kg) in 1973–81 and 1982–90. For each sex the curves in the two periods are virtually identical and describe the same pattern of faltering growth observed in earlier studies of Aborigines, as well as of many other poor populations around the world. The mean weights at a year of age were, for boys, 9.16 and 9.81 kg in the first and second periods; for girls, 8.48 and 8.85 kg, respectively. Though there appears to be an increase, there are no statistically

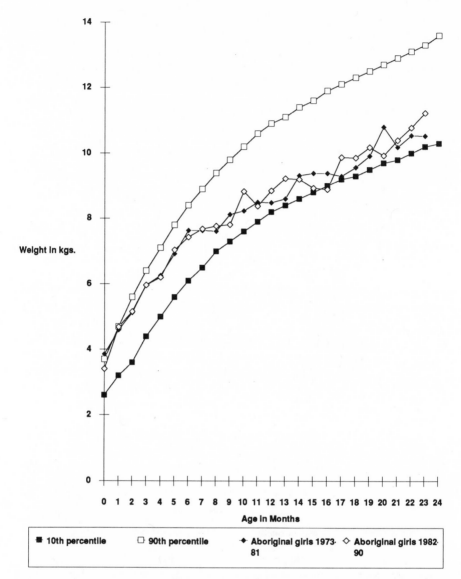

14 —

12 —

10 —

Weight in kgs.

8 —

6 —

4 —

2 —

0 —

0 1 2 3 4 5 6 7 8 9 10 11 12 13 14 15 16 17 18 19 20 21 22 23 24

Age in Months

■ 10th percentile   □ 90th percentile   ◆ Aboriginal girls 1973-
81

◇ Aboriginal girls 1982-
90

Figure 4-3   Mean weights of Aboriginal girls in 1973–81 and 1982–90, compared with Harvard standards. (*Source:* S. J. Kunitz, R. Streatfield, G. Santow, and A. de Craen, "The health of populations on North Queensland Aboriginal communities: Change and continuity," *Human Biology,* vol. 66, no. 5, 1994. Reprinted with permission of Wayne State University Press.

significant differences for boys or girls. All the average weights are slightly above or below the 30th percentile. Thus, if there has been a true increase in weight for age among infants over the past 20 years, it has not been large.

Finally, turning to life expectancy at birth, we note essentially no change over the 20-year period: for males and females combined, 57 years in 1976 and 58 in 1981 and 1986.[80] Figure 4-4 shows the life expectancies at various ages in 1976 and 1986 of Aboriginal and non-Aboriginal males and females.

It is striking how much more tightly clustered are the curves representing the experience of Aborigines than are those of non-Aborigines. This means, first, that the mortality of male and female Aborigines is much more similar than that of male and female non-Aborigines and, second, that over the decade there has been much less improvement in Aboriginal than in non-Aboriginal mortality.

The greater similarity of Aboriginal than of non-Aboriginal male and female life expectancies is not surprising. In high-mortality regimes, women tend to have higher mortality rates than men do, especially between 10 and 40 years of age, usually as a result of risks associated with childbearing. As populations experience the epidemiologic transition from high-mortality regimes dominated by infectious diseases to low-mortality regimes dominated by noninfectious conditions, women generally fare better than men do.[81] Part of the explanation has to do with reductions in fertility as well as with the increased safety of childbearing. This is not the entire explanation, however, as women have lower mortality than men do from a variety of causes, particularly including diseases of the circulatory system and injuries and poisonings. This also has been observed in various Aboriginal populations, including the Queensland communities.[82]

The widening gap between Aboriginal and non-Aboriginal life expectancies has to do with the fact that in virtually all Western European populations as well as in North America and Australia, life expectancy in adulthood has improved significantly, owing especially to an as yet unexplained decline in cardiovascular diseases since the late 1960s. Equally dramatic improvements have not occurred among Aborigines. Indeed, although there has been slight improvement, the overwhelming impression is of stagnation. Hogg and Thomson showed that in the 14 communities the observed deaths due to circulatory system diseases are between three and four times greater for Aborigines than would be expected based on rates in the non-Aboriginal population. The same is true for deaths due to injury and poisoning. The rates for men are about twice as high as those of women, and the patterns and rates have not changed for 20 years. Moreover, the ratio of age-specific death rates of Aborigines compared with non-Aborigines is especially high in the age groups of the 30s and 40s.[83] That is, it is young and early middle-aged adults who have the greatest excess mortality.

What little evidence there is suggests that mortality may not be so different between the approximately 21 to 22 percent of the Queensland Aboriginal population living in the 14 communities in northern Queensland and the remainder of the Aboriginal population of the state. For example, perinatal mortality in the 14 communities in 1988–90 was 26.9 per 1,000 live births, whereas statewide the rate for Aborigines was 30.1, for Torres Strait Islanders 26.3, and for Australian Caucasians 11.2.[84] Similarly, the life expectancies we reported for people in 12

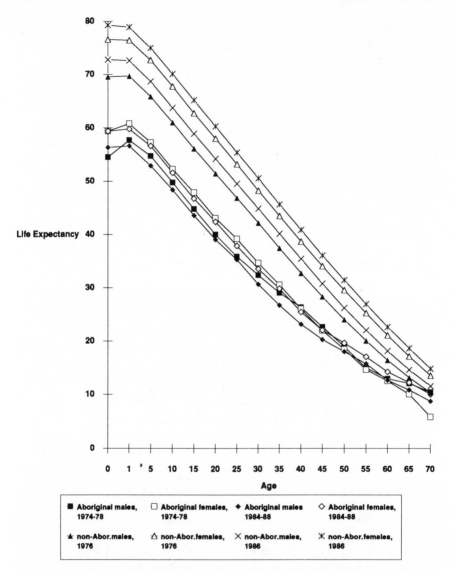

Figure 4-4 Life expectancy at various ages, male and female Aborigines and non-Aborigines, 1976 and 1986 (*Source:* S. J. Kunitz, R. Streatfield, G. Santow, and A. de Craen, "The health of populations on North Queensland Aboriginal communities: Change and continuity," *Human Biology,* vol. 66, no. 5, 1994. Reprinted with permission of Wayne State University Press.

of the communities were similar to the intercensal estimates calculated by Alan Gray for the entire Aboriginal population of the state. For males in the 12 communities the life expectancy was about 56 years at birth in 1986 and 60 for females, compared with statewide figures of 55.8 for males and 64.0 for females.[85] Thus females in the communities have a lower life expectancy than do females elsewhere, but males have about the same. On the other hand, in the 3 years 1990 through 1992 there was a total of 38 homicides in which Aborigines were the victims, and of these almost half (18) were from the communities. Therefore the homicide rate is higher in the communities than elsewhere in the state.[86]

In general these data suggest that with the exception of infant mortality, the health of the Aborigines in Queensland has not improved substantially in the past 20 years, despite increasing expenditures by both the federal and state governments. Part of the explanation surely has to do with the fact that preventive and curative services have been fragmented; that the health problems associated with mental disorders and alcohol abuse have not been adequately addressed, even though they were recognized two decades ago; and that until recently the extraordinarily high rates of death from cardiovascular diseases have not even begun to attract the attention they deserve. This fragmentation can be attributed to the different ways in which health problems and the provision of services have been understood by various interested parties, to their different political agendas, and to the Australian federal structure that has made possible the proliferation of competing interest groups in Aboriginal health.

THE AGE OF REFORM

Historical periods, like most categories, are fuzzy, particularly the closer they are to the observer. The late 1980s and early 1990s were no exception. In 1987 two entities were created that have had an enormous impact on Aboriginal health policy in Queensland, although only time will tell whether they will truly form a watershed between two historical periods. The first, created by the Queensland state government, was the Commission of Inquiry into Possible Illegal Activities and Associated Police Misconduct, more often known as the Fitzgerald Inquiry, after the chairman of the commission. The second was the National Aboriginal Health Strategy Working Party, which was agreed on at a meeting in December 1987 of commonwealth, state, and territory ministers responsible for health and Aboriginal affairs.

The Fitzgerald Inquiry resulted from stories in the press and on television in 1987 of police corruption in Queensland. Such stories had surfaced before but had always been denied and never became the subject of an official inquiry. This time, however, Premier Bjelke-Petersen was campaigning for the office of prime minister, and his deputy premier was left in control while his attention was elsewhere. For reasons that have been the subject of some speculation, a commission of inquiry was created and supported by the state government.[87] It soon became clear, as Fitzgerald wrote, "that police corruption was widespread, and part of a bigger problem."[88] That problem had to do with the political culture that had developed in Queensland over the course of the century. It was a culture of secrecy, in which the separation of powers had been ignored or forgotten, in which the gerrymander had been used shamelessly to retain control of government, in which individual gain from political office was routine, in which political decisions influenced not only policy but also the administration of policy, and in which civil liberties were abused. Fitzgerald continued: "This Commission of

Inquiry commenced with very limited terms of reference which expanded greatly. It began by pulling a few threads at the frayed edges of society. To general
alarm, sections of the fabric began to unravel."[89]

The pervasiveness of corruption could no longer be ignored, especially after a
number of major political figures went to jail. The result was that in 1989 the
Labor party won control of the state government for the first time since 1957.
The new premier, Wayne Goss, wrote:

> Since the late 1980s, arising mainly from the Fitzgerald inquiry and its aftermath, the
> Queensland public sector has been undergoing major changes to strengthen the integrity
> with which government business is handled, to improve efficiency, and to provide
> better service to the people of Queensland. . . .
> Radical overhaul of the public sector as part of the reform process was specifically
> given high priority by the Goss Government upon its election in December 1989.
> The public sector in Queensland is composed of many experienced people committed
> to serving the Queensland community. Despite this, it has historically been a public
> sector impeded in its capacity to provide quality performance by organizational frag-
> mentation, an absence of policy mechanisms, over-centralised decision-making and
> excessive concentration of senior staff in Brisbane. It was also a public sector with little
> interest in fostering the talent and abilities of its staff, or, except at the most junior
> levels, in attracting talented and able people.[90]

The document went on to say that "the 1990s is notable for the emphasis on
public accountability" and that "this would have a major bearing on how organizations perform their work."[91] In the Department of Health this meant regionalization and decentralization. The director-general of the Health Department
wrote:

> The *Health Services Act (1991)*, which abolished Queensland's 59 Hospital Boards,
> represented the most far-reaching change to Queensland's health system in more than
> 50 years. It resulted in a move away from a centralised administrative system to a
> regionalised public sector health service system which can be more responsive to local
> community and client needs.[92]

Coincidentally, the final report of the National Aboriginal Health Strategy
Working Party was released in March 1989.[93] The meeting that had led to the
creation of the working party had been concerned with creating a national policy
for Aboriginal health. In a discussion paper presented to the meeting, it had been
observed that among the constraints on the development of such a policy in the
past was the fact that "Commonwealth/State relations have not always been
smooth due to differing political philosophies and sensitivities. Poorly defined
responsibilities have resulted in an unco-ordinated approach to Aboriginal health
care."[94] Among the Working Party's many recommendations were that there be
established tripartite forums that would include representatives of the commonwealth and state governments as well as representatives of Aboriginal community organizations involved in health. Such forums would address questions
about intersectoral collaboration on health matters; the implications of devolving

decision making and control to local levels; the adequacy of integration among preventive, curative, and rehabilitative services; and the effectiveness of referral processes among primary, secondary, and tertiary levels of care.[95]

Clearly this was an attempt to integrate the policies of various levels of government as well as to be responsive to the organizations that represented Aboriginal consumers of health services. Coming as it did just as a new Queensland government had achieved power with a mandate for reform and increased public accountability, the Working Party's recommendations were largely accepted as the guide for the state's Aboriginal health policy. This included disbanding the Aboriginal Health Program, dispersing its workers to the new regional offices, and creating in its place an Aboriginal Health Policy Unit in the central office in Brisbane. A major goal of the unit is "to facilitate the development of culturally valid and technically sound health strategies for the Aborigines and Torres Strait Islanders in Queensland."[96] This is to be done in a variety of ways, one of which is to encourage and foster liaison with a variety of Aboriginal organizations and communities:

There is a need for existing representative, advocacy and consultative structures to address issues which currently impede the participation of indigenous people in all aspects of the health system. Indigenous people have the right to take part in decision making processes which affect their health, and to do so in a manner consistent with indigenous cultural protocols. This participation must encompass health services both within and outside the mainstream health system.[97]

In 1989, the same year that Labor came to power in Queensland and the National Aboriginal Health Strategy was released, there was another significant development: The commonwealth government's Department of Aboriginal Affairs was changed to the Aboriginal and Torres Strait Islander Commission (ATSIC). It was organized on a decentralized basis, with the central office creating policy guidelines but having no line authority for implementing policy. Indeed, regional councils, all composed of Aborigines and Islanders elected from the regions, have the final decision-making authority over how the funds allocated to their regions are to be spent. Since these monies are to be spent on health and many other activities (roads, housing, etc.), each of the regions may divide up its resources in different ways. As with the regionalization of the Queensland Health Department, it is still too early to know what the consequences of this development will be.

For my purposes, what is important is that these changes represent major shifts in both state and commonwealth government Aboriginal health policy: devolution from strongly entrenched central control to regional centers, from confrontation to at least an attempt at rapprochement, and from professional dominance to lay influence. What is not yet clear is whether these changes will lead to improved health, whether they are simply cosmetic, and whether the fragmentation that has characterized the past will dominate the future as well. That reform is taking place seems clear. Whether a Reformation has occurred is still far from certain.

CONCLUSIONS

The purpose of this chapter has been to make two points. First, throughout the 19th century in Queensland it was not diseases acting independently that reduced the population but the conscious slaughter of Aborigines on a massive scale, the destruction of the environments on which they depended, starvation, and disease. The magnitude of the decline was appalling, as it was for many indigenous peoples, but it was not disease alone that was responsible. Slaughter on such a grand scale did not occur in Hawaii and New Zealand, where social and economic dislocation, crowding, and malnutrition seem to have been relatively more important.

Second, the failure of Aboriginal life expectancy and health in general to improve as significantly as it has among North American Indians and Maoris is due largely to the fact that for most of the past 200 years it has been first the colonies and then their successor states or territories that have been charged with responsibility for Aboriginal affairs. As I argued in Chapter 2, this has been particularly detrimental to Aborigines' interests because of the close relationship that ranchers, miners, and others have had to the state governments. The examples of Mapoon, Weipa, and Aurukun in Queensland all illustrate the point. This also explains the unwillingness of the state government to be generous in its provision of special services, and its insistence that Aborigines have, and should exercise, the same rights of access to the health care system as other citizens have.

This legacy has complicated attempts by the commonwealth government to intervene in Aboriginal health conditions because states continue to have vested rights in Aboriginal affairs, particularly those pertaining to land. The result has been that when the commonwealth did intervene, conflict erupted; services proliferated in an uncoordinated and fragmented fashion; many health needs were not addressed; and there were no substantial improvements in health.

Adding to these complications is the fact that the relationships between the commonwealth and state governments and Aboriginal organizations have never been congenial. Commonwealth–state relationships are complicated by party affiliations and by changing policies when governments change hands. Commonwealth relations with Aboriginal medical services are complicated by distrust and demands for accountability on the part of the government and resentment of inadequate funding and attempted control on the side of the medical services. And of course, state health departments and Aboriginal medical services have been in competition for the same pots of commonwealth money.

These different positions are reflected in different ways of defining health and disease, evaluating services, and understanding what is valid knowledge and professional expertise. As exemplified by the material from Queensland, spokemen for State Health Departments have tended to see themselves as commanding professional expertise. Their notion of health is usually not defined but seems to be confined to the presence or absence of diagnosable or measurable conditions. Their understanding of their tasks tends to be circumscribed and well defined (e.g., reducing acute malnutrition and infant mortality), and the interventions equally circumscribed. Even though they may recognize the significance of the larger context, it is thought to be beyond their area of responsibility. Professional expertise is viewed as central to defining the goals of programs, and hard end-points (e.g., death rates, prevalence of various conditions) are the measure of success or failure.

The Aboriginal medical services and their supporters differ on every point. They generally accept the World Health Organization's definition of health as complete physical, mental, and social well-being. This means that everything influences health, and hence the task of providers of services is equally broad and may involve various forms of advocacy and political action. Because the definition of health and of the professional task is so encompassing, the achievement of good health means the participation of far more than professionally trained experts. Moreover, participation in meaningful work is in itself thought to promote good health, and therefore outcome measures are often "soft" and processual rather than "hard." Thus involvement by community members in making and implementing policy is in itself considered to be health promoting, regardless even of the consequences of the policy in regard to, say, mortality rates.[98] For example, a review of an Aboriginal community health service states:

Aboriginal culture is the very antithesis of Western ideology. The accent on individual commitment, the concept of linear time, the switch in focus from spiritual to worldly, the emphasis on possession and the pricing of goods and services, the rape of the environment and, above all, the devaluing of relationships between people, both within families and within the whole community, as the determinant of social behaviour, are totally at variance with the fundamental belief system of Aboriginal people.

"Health" to Aboriginal peoples is a matter of determining all aspects of their life, including control over their physical environment, of dignity, of community self-esteem, and of justice. It is not merely a matter of the provision of doctors, hospitals, medicines or the absence of disease and incapacity. . . .

Aboriginal medicine seeks to provide a meaningful explanation for illness and to respond to the personal, family, and community issues surrounding illness have survived [sic]. Aboriginal medicine and practices are a complex system closely linked to land based cultural beliefs. For this reason, Aborigines in contemporary Australia see health as a sovereign issue. . . .

This Working Party therefore see health as:

"Not just the physical well-being of the individual but the social, emotional, and cultural well-being of the whole community. This is a whole-of-life view and it also includes the cyclical concept of life–death–life."

Our working definition of primary health care is:

"Essential health care based on practical, scientifically sound, socially and culturally acceptable methods and technology made universally accessible to individuals and families in the communities in which they live through their full participation at every stage of development in the spirit of self-reliance and self-determination."[99]

I have stated these positions baldly but, I think, fairly. They are in fact characterizations of what are usually called vertical and horizontal health programs. An example of the former is the disease eradication campaigns such as those aimed at smallpox and malaria. An example of the latter is the primary care program advocated by the signatories of the Declaration of Alma-Ata, the WHO–UNICEF document that is so often cited by people working in Aboriginal medical services.[100]

Predictably, the two sides have little use for each other. I have already given some indications of the State Health Department's views. In response, Minister for Aboriginal Affairs R. I. Viner wrote:

> The view which is now increasingly advanced by the Sates, that Aboriginal involvement in planning, management and control is inimical to the responsibilities and expertise of health professionals, seems to me to be unnecessarily rigid and indicative of an inadequate response to the continuing low health status of Aboriginals and their determination to change it. This resistance to acknowledgment of real community responsibilities, and reliance on more conventional service bases has led to underutilised facilities for which professional staffing was scarce or unavailable and an undue reliance on Aboriginal health workers for community input.[101]

Advocates for Aboriginal medical services have said something similar. For instance, the Queensland representative to the conference of Australian health ministers in 1988 tabled a recommendation "that Commonwealth funded, State-delivered Aboriginal Health Programs which are already acknowledged as effective, continue to receive Commonwealth financial support without reduction." The reasons given were

> It would be inappropriate to place a complex Health Program in the hands of an Aboriginal or any other interest group even if it is representative of the target population.
>
> To transfer such funds . . . in the name of Aboriginal Control, into the hands of organisations lacking much professional expertise would be a retrograde and irresponsible step.

In response, Moodie wrote, "These comments not only reflect lack of understanding of how community-controlled health services work but also reflect an institutionalised, bureaucratised form of racism."[102]

Both horizontal and vertical programs have much to be said for them. The eradication of smallpox has been a remarkable achievement. The reduction of other vaccine-preventable diseases has also avoided much suffering. But on the other hand, as the Queensland example suggests, the failure to address major psychosocial influences on health and well-being has resulted in the stagnation of several (hard) measures of mortality and morbidity. This was not simply because of bureaucratic fragmentation but because only late in the day did the state program begin to take these problems seriously.

Community-controlled horizontal programs, on the other hand, are more likely to attend to what the consumers of their services have to say, and the evidence suggests that they were thus more attuned earlier to the significance of psychosocial problems such as substance abuse and its dire consequences for individuals, families, and entire communities. On the other hand, the broad definition of health, and the view that everything causes everything else, can result in rhetoric that strains even the most generous notions of cause and effect. For example, a submission to the National Aboriginal Health Strategy Working Party from the Victorian Aboriginal Health Services stated:

> Sovereignty IS self-determination for Aboriginal peoples. By definition, this includes the final say in the management of our economic, social, cultural, and political resources. Sovereignty will allow us to tie resources to community needs in one move, independent of political or bureaucratic interference or threat thereof.
>
> "Big brother" not trusting us, looking over our shoulder breeds distrust, resentment, and unaccountability. Accountability of Aboriginal people to their own communities, however, will lead to a restoration of traditional structures and traditional values. Community initiative, community participation, and community control are the tools for implementing sovereignty.
>
> In the context of a national health strategy, sovereignty is a practical response to Aboriginal needs in the areas of housing, education, employment, health, legal and judicial systems, child care, and care of the elderly. In addition, sovereignty is an appropriate response to the complex causative factors underlying Aboriginal deaths in custody.[103]

It is clear that the official spokesmen for the Queensland State Health Department have for 60 years enunciated policies regarding Aboriginal health that were consistent with the political culture and economic goals of the state government. Indeed, it was their association with the state that gave them legitimacy. In turn, their professional expertise worked to legitimize state policy.

Community-based organizations also derive their legitimacy from state institutions. Their legitimating ideology is drawn from WHO's definition of health, produced by professional public health workers and psychiatrists shortly after World War II; from the Declaration of Alma-Ata, produced by WHO and UNICEF health professionals from the poor countries of the South intent on extracting more aid from the rich countries of the North; and from notions of self-determination, produced by professional diplomats in the League of Nations and the United Nations. These ideas find their institutional expression in "community-based" organizations that are dependent on commonwealth support for their continuing viability. In this case the ideology of the professionals requires the existence of communities.

The reality is more complex. As Maggie Brady wrote:

> Aboriginal communities are rarely communal, having been thrown together, at least in remote Australia, as a result of historical and administrative expediency. Even in groups of people who share the same language and social organization, and who have lived together for fifty years or more, cohesive "communalism" is non-existent. . . . While the uncritical and bland use of the term "community" continues, with its concomitant allusions to homogeneity, communalism and collective decision-making, policy decisions and intervention programs . . . can go badly askew.[104]

And in respect of a small Aboriginal community on the Cape York Peninsula, Christopher Anderson noted:

> The problem with this "community" was two-fold: One, people were under virtual compulsion to live here under the old Queensland *Aborigines Act*. As I have noted, although homogeneous at one level, Wujalwujal contains groups from different areas— "mobs" associated with the old permanent camps—and who are at constant odds with each other; the council structure which was eventually set up was wholly dominated by one group; community living was tense, close and difficult; the unequal economic and political status between groups was stark and easily apparent. Second, a community such as Wujalwujal with its population of over 300 people has little hope of ever becoming in any way self-sufficient with its present concentrated land base . . . It is totally artificial in economic terms.
>
> In order to really exist (i.e. the management by individuals and families of their own lives), the community has to disband; in order to get continuing funds from the State, it must prove that it *is* a community (and go along with policies such as self-management). In other words, they have to continue the very conditions which lead to the problems. "Self-management" and "community" are here contradiction in terms (italics in original).[105]

The point is, simply, that the ideology of "community control," "community self-management," and "self-determination" is a professional ideology based on positions enunciated by professional experts; it draws its institutional support from government; and it derives its legitimacy from the existence of "communities." Where communities do not exist, they must be invented. And where community conflict and factionalism exist, they are said to be an internalization of government conflicts, not a feature of Aboriginal social organization, which is exacerbated by the creation of spurious communities by the coercive power of the state.

It seems to me inevitable and usually productive that there are such contending professional ideologies of health and the role of health workers. It is inevitable because political ideals and aspirations differ, institutional locations differ, and economic interests differ. It is potentially productive because, as my examples were meant to suggest, both positions have admirable strengths as well as appalling weaknesses. Out of the debates between adherents to each may come more adequate solutions than either would produce if left unchecked. Unhappily, in the Australian system of federalism in regard to Aboriginal affairs, the conflict so far has been institutionalized at such a high intensity that the result has been unproductive, for Aboriginal health has failed to improve substantially.

NOTES

1. R. Fitzgerald, *A History of Queensland from the Dreaming to 1915* (St. Lucia: University of Queensland Press, 1982), p. 135.

2. N. Loos, *Invasion and Resistance: Aboriginal–European Relations on the North Queensland Frontier 1861–1897* (Canberra: Australian National University Press, 1982), p. 31.

3. C. D. Rowley, *The Destruction of Aboriginal Society: Aboriginal Policy and Practice—Volume I* (Canberra: Australian National University Press, 1970), p. 152.

4. R. Evans, K. Saunders, and K. Cronin, *Race Relations in Colonial Queensland: A History of Exclusion, Exploitation and Extermination* (St. Lucia: University of Queensland Press, 1975), p. 51.

5. Loos, *Invasion and Resistance,* pp. 68–69.

6. Ibid., p. 79.

7. Ibid., pp. 103–5. See also C. Anderson, "Queensland Aboriginal peoples today," in J. H. Holmes, ed., *Queensland, a Geographical Interpretation,* Queensland Geographical Journal, 4th series, vol. 1, 1986, p. 302.

8. Loos, *Invasion and Resistance,* pp. 149–53. See also N. Sharp, *Footprints Along the Cape York Sandbeaches* (Canberra: Aboriginal Studies Press, 1992).

9. Loos, *Invasion and Resistance,* p. 142.

10. A Chase, "Which way now? Tradition, continuity and change in a North Queensland Aboriginal community" (Ph.D. diss., University of Queensland, 1980), pp. 371–72. A similar situation has been described at Bloomfield River in the southeast Cape York Peninsula. (J.) C. Anderson, "The political and economic basis of Kuku-Yalanji social history," (Ph.D. diss., University of Queensland, 1984).

11. D. May, "The articulation of the Aboriginal and capitalist modes on the North Queensland pastoral frontier," *Journal of Australian Studies* 12(1983):34–44.

12. Rowley, *The Destruction of Aboriginal Society,* p. 167.

13. Ibid., p. 302.

14. Ibid., p. 167.

15. Loos, *Invasion and Resistance,* pp. 165–67. H. Wearne, *A Clash of Cultures: Queensland Aboriginal Policy (1824–1980)* (Brisbane: Division of World Mission of the Uniting Church of Australia, 1980), p. 9.

16. Loos, *Invasion and Resistance,* p. 174; N. Loos, "Concern and contempt: Church and missionary attitudes towards Aborigines in North Queensland in the nineteenth century," in T. Swain and D. B. Rose, eds., *Aboriginal Australians and Christian Missions: Ethnographic and Historical Studies* (Bedford, S.A.: Australian Association for the Study of Religions, 1988), p. 111. According to Ken Inglis (personal communication), J. L. Stokes said in 1846: "To smooth, as it were, the pillow of an expiring peoples." The phrase was repeated in *The Age* (Melbourne), October 28, 1858. Later writers seem to have mistaken *smooth* for *soothe.*

17. Rowley, *The Destruction of Aboriginal Society,* p. 180.

18. Wearne, *A Clash of Cultures,* p. 12.

19. R. W. Cilento, *The White Man in the Tropics: With Especial Reference to Australia and Its Dependencies* (Melbourne: H. J. Green, Government Printer, 1925), pp. 90–91.

20. R. W. Cilento, *Interim Report on Aboriginals—Survey no. 1* (October–November 1932), Australian Archives, no. A1928/1, 4/5 sec. 1, p. 4.

21. Ibid., p. 21.

22. L. Lippmann, *Generations of Resistance: Aborigines Demand Justice* (Melbourne: Longman Cheshire, 1991), p. 24.

23. Wearne, *A Clash of Cultures,* p. 14.

24. D. May, *The health of Aborigines on North Queensland cattle stations,"* in R. MacLeod and D. Denoon, eds., *Health and Healing in Tropical Australia and Papua New Guinea* (Townsville, Qld.: James Cook University, 1991), pp. 129–30; D. May, "Early health problems in Aboriginals," in J. Pearn, ed., *Pioneer Medicine in Australia* (Brisbane: Amphion Press, 1988), pp. 175–184. D. May, "Race relations in Queensland 1897–1971," in Commissioner L. F. Wyvill, Q. C., "Royal Commission into Aboriginal deaths

in custody," *Regional Report of Inquiry in Queensland,* app. 1(b) (Canberra: Australian Government Publishing Service, 1991), pp. 137–38. See also D. S. Trigger, *Whitefella Comin': Aboriginal Responses to Colonialism in Northern Australia* (Cambridge: Cambridge University Press, 1992), p. 59.

25. Cilento, *Interim Report no. 1,* p. 2.

26. Ibid., pp. 2–3. South Sea Islanders—so-called Kanakas—had been employed to work on sugar plantations in Queensland. The White Australia policy had as one of its objects the exclusion of such workers. In return for the loss of these low-paid workers, sugar planters were assured high prices in a protected domestic market.

27. B. Rosser, *Dreamtime Nightmares: Biographies of Aborigines Under the Queensland Aborigines Act* (Canberra: Australian Institute of Aboriginal Studies, 1985).

28. Director of Native Affairs, *Annual Reports* (Brisbane: Government Printer, various years).

29. Lippmann, *Generations of Resistance,* p. 27.

30. Wearne, *A Clash of Cultures,* p. 16.

31. R. Fitzgerald, *A History of Queensland from 1915 to the 1980s* (St. Lucia: University of Queensland Press, 1985), chap. 7. See also P. Wilson, *Black Death, White Hands* (North Sydney: Allen & Unwin, 1985), F. Brennan, *Land Rights Queensland Style: The Struggle for Aboriginal Self-Management* (St. Lucia: University of Queensland Press, 1992).

32. W. J. Fysh, R. Davison, D. Chandler, and A. E. Dugdale, "The weights of Aboriginal infants: A comparison over 20 years," *Medical Journal of Australia,* June 4, 1977, pp. 13–15.

33. D. G. Jose, M. H. R. Self, and N. D. Stallman, "A survey of children and adolescents on Queensland Aboriginal settlements, 1967," *Australian Paediatric Journal* 5(1969):71–88; D. G. Jose and J. S. Welch, "Growth retardation, anaemia and infection, with malabsorption and infestation of the bowel: The syndrome of protein-calorie malnutrition in Australian Aboriginal children," *Medical Journal of Australia* 1(1970):349–56.

34. Jose and Welsh, "Growth retardation," p. 350.

35. Ibid., p. 349.

36. Lippmann, *Generations of Resistance,* p. 32.

37. S. Bennett, "The 1967 referendum," *Australian Aboriginal Studies,* no. 2 (1985):26–31.

38. S. Bennett, "Federalism and Aboriginal affairs," *Australian Aboriginal Studies,* no. 1 (1988):18–27.

39. W. Sanders, *Aboriginal affairs,"* in B. Galligan, O. Hughes, and C. Walsh, eds., *Intergovernmental Relations and Public Policy* (Sydney: Allen & Unwin, 1991), pp. 257–76.

40. C. Fletcher, *Aboriginal Politics: Intergovernmental Relations* (Melbourne: Melbourne University Press, 1992), p. 8.

41. See, for instance, G. Nettheim, *Victims of the Law: Black Queenslanders Today* (Sydney: Allen & Unwin, 1981), pp. 10–14. The story is told most powerfully from the point of view of the people at Aurukun in a film made at the time: *Takeover,* directed by David MacDougall and Judith MacDougall (Canberra: Australian Institute of Aboriginal Studies, released 1980).

42. Jose et al., "A survey of children"; Jose and Welch, "Growth retardation," 1970.

43. S. J. Kunitz, "Explanations of ideologies of mortality declines," *Population and Development Review* 13(1987):379–408.

44. I. A. Musgrave, *Report on Health of Mainland Aborigines in Queensland Resulting from a Survey of the Mainland Aboriginal Communities and Reserves over the Period 12 May to 27th November, 1970* (Brisbane: Queensland Department of Health, 1970).

45. Ibid.

46. M. T. Samisoni and J. I. Samisoni, "The health of Aboriginal and Islander children in urbanized communities," *Australian Nurses' Journal* 7(1978):44–47.

47. A. K. Eckermann, "Half-caste, out-caste: An ethnographic analysis of the processes underlying adaptation among Aboriginal people in rural town, south-west Queensland" (Ph.D. diss., University of Queensland, 1977), p. 380.

48. Ibid., p. 381.

49. A. Eckermann, T. Dowd, M. Martin, L. Nixon, R. Gray, and E. Chong, *Binanj Goonj: Bridging Cultures in Aboriginal Health* (Armidale, N.S.W.: University of New England, 1992), pp. 64–65.

50. I. A. Musgrave, *A Chronicle of the Aboriginal Health Program Including a Profile of Some Major Aspects of the Health of Aborigines in Queensland and Showing Trends in the 5 Years 1972–76* (Brisbane: Queensland Department of Health, 1977), p. 135.

51. Musgrave, *Report*, p. 88.

52. Ibid., p. 89. Award wages are wages agreed on by collective bargaining. Historically, Aboriginal workers were not included in such settlements and were often paid a fraction of what white workers were paid for the same work. Work on communities was also paid at much lower rates than elsewhere.

53. Ibid., p. 91.

54. Ibid., p. 92. "Assisted Aborigines" were people who even as late as 1970 still had their affairs controlled by Queensland's Department of Aboriginal and Islander Affairs.

55. For example, see the comments a few years later by A. E. Dugdale in his testimony before the House of Representatives (Reps) Standing Committee on Aboriginal Affairs (Aboriginal Health), Brisbane, July 7, 1978. Some informants say that hospital nurses employed by the State Department of Aboriginal and Islander Affairs (which ran most of the hospitals in the Queensland communities) would not cooperate with public health nurses working in the same communities and employed by the health department after the establishment of the Aboriginal Health Program in 1972.

56. W. Sanders, "From self-determination to self-management," in P. Loveday, ed., *Service Delivery to Remote Communities* (Darwin: Australian National University North Australia Research Unit, 1982), pp. 4–10.

57. R. I. Viner, *Submission by the Minister for Aboriginal Affairs,* Reps (House of Representatives) Standing Committee on Aboriginal Affairs, Aboriginal Health, Canberra, November 10, 1978, p. 4406.

58. Ibid., p. 4407.

59. R. Patrick, *A History of Health and Medicine in Queensland 1824–1960* (St. Lucia: University of Queensland Press, 1987), esp. app. E, "Queensland's Free Hospital Scheme"; G. Lewis, "Queensland nationalism and Australian capitalism," in E. L. Wheelwright and K. Buckley, eds., *Essays in the Political Economy of Australian Capitalism* (Sydney: Australia and New Zealand Book Company, 1978), vol. 2, p. 122.

60. I. A. Musgrave, *Supplement to Chronicles of the Aboriginal Health Programme, Now Encompassing the 6 Years 1972–1977* (Brisbane: Queensland Department of Health, 1978), pp. 18–19.

61. Nettheim, *Victims of the Law,* pp. 21–22.

62. Quoted from ibid., p. 23.

63. Letter of September 2, 1982, from Ian Wilson, Minister for Aboriginal Affairs (Canberra), to K. B. Tomkins, Minister for Water Resources and Aboriginal and Island Affairs, Brisbane, file 1000–0023-002 (Brisbane: Queensland Department of Health).

64. R. P. Davison, Director of the Aboriginal Health Program, "Briefing paper for the minister for health on the proposed withdrawal of ATSIC funding for AHP," November 22, 1990, file 1000-0023-011 (Brisbane: Queensland Department of Health). ATSIC is

the acronym for the Aboriginal and Torres Strait Islander Commission, the successor agency to the federal Department of Aboriginal Affairs.

65. "Notes of meeting, Department of Health/Department of Aboriginal and Islanders Advancement," May 13, 1981, file 1000-0023-002 (Brisbane: Queensland Department of Health). The Department of Aboriginal and Islanders Advancement was the new name of the state's Department of Aboriginal and Islanders Affairs.

66. R. Moodie, "The politics of evaluating Aboriginal health services," *Community Health Studies* 13(1989):503–9.

67. I. A. Musgrave, *Submission to the Reps Standing Committee on Aboriginal Affairs* (Aboriginal Health), Brisbane, July 7, 1978, p. 1868.

68. Human Rights and Equal Opportunity Commission, *The Provision of Health and Medical Services to the Aboriginal Communities of Cooktown, Hopevale and Wujal Wujal* (Sydney, 1991), p. 55.

69. I. A. Musgrave, *Submission*, p. 1956.

70. R. Speare and K. A. Kelly, *Health Needs of Aboriginals and Islanders in the Townsville Region: The Role of Black Medical Services* (Townsville, Qld.: Anton Breinl Centre for Tropical Health and Medicine, James Cook University, 1991).

71. J. P. Reser and S. A. Morrissey, *Aboriginal Mental Health and Mental Health Services in Queensland: Fragmented and Forgotten,* Consultant's Report to the Rights and Culture Branch of the Department of Family Services and Aboriginal and Torres Strait Islander Affairs (Townsville, Qld.: James Cook University of North Queensland, 1991), pp. 54–55.

72. R. Davison, *An Analysis of All Health Services Currently Provided to the Aboriginal and Torres Strait Islander Citizens of Queensland* (Brisbane: Aboriginal Health Program, Queensland Department of Health, 1990), pp. 18–19.

73. Ibid., p. 32.

74. Ibid., p. 28.

75. R. Hogg and N. Thomson, *Fertility and Mortality of Aborigines Living in the Queensland Aboriginal Communities 1972–1990,* Aboriginal and Torres Strait Islander Health Series no. 8 (Canberra: Australian Institute of Health and Welfare, 1992), p. 10.

76. *Perinatal Statistics, Queensland 1987* and *Queensland 1988* (Brisbane: Epidemiology and Health Information Branch, Queensland Department of Health, 1990 and 1991).

77. The following discussions of growth and of life expectancy and Figures 4-2, 4-3, and 4-4 are from S. J. Kunitz, R. Streatfield, G. Santow, and A. de Craen, "The health of populations on North Queensland Aboriginal communities: Change and continuity," *Human Biology,* vol. 6, no. 5, 1994.

78. J. W. Cox, "A longitudinal study of the changing pattern in Aboriginal infants' growth 1966–76," *Journal of Biosocial Science* 11(1979):269–79.

79. J. W. Cox, "Growth characteristics of preschool Aboriginal children," *Australian Paediatric Journal* 15(1979):10–15.

80. These figures are based on data from 12 North Queensland Aboriginal communities. The details are in Kunitz et al., "The health of populations." These estimates of life expectancy at birth are higher than those calculated by Hogg and Thomson, *Fertility and Mortality,* using data from the same 12 communities on which our estimates were based, plus two others. We think the discrepancy is due to the fact that they did not adjust for the underenumeration of children. Our figures are consistent with estimates made elsewhere by N. Thomson and N. Briscoe, *Overview of Aboriginal Health Status in Queensland,* Aboriginal and Torres Strait Islander Health Series no. 4 (Canberra: Australian Institute of

Health, 1991). They are also consistent with intercensal survival estimates made by Alan Gray for each state and the Northern Territory. Published in N. Thomson, "A review of Aboriginal health status," in J. Reid and P. Trompf, eds., *The Health of Aboriginal Australia* (Sydney: Harcourt Brace Jovanovich, 1991), p. 45.

81. A. R. Omran, "The epidemiologic transition," *Milbank Memorial Fund Quarterly* 49(1971):509–38.

82. Hogg and Thomson, *Fertility and Mortality,* p. 17.

83. Ibid., pp. 15–17.

84. *Perinatal Statistics, Queensland 1988,* p. 53.

85. The intercensal estimates are cited in N. Thomson, "A review of Aboriginal health status," p. 45.

86. The homicide data were made available by Heather Strang, Australian Institute of Criminology, Canberra. For a description of the data sources and more discussion of rates and patterns, see H. Strang, *Homicides in Australia 1989–90* and *Homicides in Australia 1990–91* (Canberra: Australian Institute of Criminology, 1991 and 1992). See also D. F. Martin, "Aboriginal and non-Aboriginal homicide: 'Same but different,'" in H. Strang and S-A Gerull, *Homicide: Patterns, Prevention and Control* (Canberra: Australian Institute of Criminology, 1993), pp. 167–76.

87. Commission of Inquiry into Possible Illegal Activities and Associated Police Misconduct, *Report of a Commission of Inquiry Pursuant to Orders in Council* (Brisbane: Government Printer, 1989). See also P. Coaldrake, *Working the System: Government in Queensland* (St. Lucia: University of Queensland Press, 1989); P. Dicking, *The Road to Fitzgerald and Beyond* (St. Lucia: University of Queensland Press, 1988).

88. Commission of Inquiry, *Report,* p. 3.

89. Ibid., p. 4.

90. W. Goss, "Foreword," in *Managing Queensland's Public Sector* (Brisbane: Public Sector Management Commission, 1992), p. 1.

91. Ibid., p. 3.

92. P. H. Stanley, "Director General's Message," in *Corporate Plan 1992–97* (Brisbane: Queensland Health, 1992), p. 4.

93. National Aboriginal Health Strategy Working Party, *A National Aboriginal Health Strategy,* 1989.

94. Anon. "Process for development of a national policy on Aboriginal health," discussion paper presented to the commonwealth, state, and territory ministers responsible for health and Aboriginal affairs, December 1987, file 1000-0023,007 (Brisbane: Queensland Department of Health).

95. National Aboriginal Health Strategy Working Party, *Strategy,* pp. 38–39.

96. Aboriginal Health Policy Unit, "Towards the development of a Queensland Aboriginal and Torres Strait Islander health policy," background issues paper (Brisbane: Queensland Department of Health, 1993), p. 15.

97. Ibid., p. 25.

98. I. Anderson, *Koorie Health in Koorie Hands* (Melbourne: Koorie Health Unit, Health Department, Victoria, 1988), p. 137.

99. B. Bartlett, D. Legge, and D. Scrimgeour, *Anyinginyi Congress: A Vision for Aboriginal Health,* Report of a review commissioned by the Aboriginal and Torres Strait Islander Commission (ATSIC) on behalf of ATSIC and the Anyinginyi Congress Aboriginal Corporation (Tennant Creek) and conducted in December 1991 (February 1992 [no place of publication listed]), pp. 111–12.

100. Kunitz, "Explanations of Ideologies."

101. Viner, *Submission*, p. 4408.

102. Moodie, "The politics of evaluating," p. 506. See also S. Saggers and D. Gray, *Aboriginal Health and Society: The Traditional and Contemporary Aboriginal Struggle for Better Health* (Sydney: Allen & Unwin, 1991), pp. 154–56.

103. Victorian Aboriginal Health Services Co-Op Ltd., "Land rights, sovereignty and health," *Aboriginal and Islander Health Worker* 14(1990):12–13. See also National Aboriginal Health Strategy Working Party, *Strategy*, pp. ix–xi.

104. M. Brady, "Barriers to effective intervention in Aboriginal substance abuse," paper presented at the Annual Conference of the Public Health Association of Australia, Alice Springs, N.T., September 29–October 2, 1991, pp. 11–12.

105. C. Anderson, "Deaths in custody: Kuku-Yalanji and the state," *Social Analysis* 31(1992):8–9.

5

The Impact of Sociocultural Differences
on Health

Previous chapters have emphasized the powerful impact that national and subnational levels of government have had on the health of the indigenous peoples of Northern America, Polynesia, and Australia. In this and the next chapter we return to the comparative method. Our focus shifts, however, to the importance of indigenous cultures for the health of their members. Our examples are the Hopi and Navajo Indians in the Southwest of the United States, chosen because they live in the same environment; have been coerced by the same government in similar ways (e.g., in regard to forced education and stock reduction in the 1930s); have been forced to acquiesce in the extraction of their natural resources in the interests of the same large corporation (e.g., the Peabody Coal Company, which operates a large strip mine on land claimed by both tribes); and are beneficiaries of the same health, education, and welfare systems.[1] Yet they have very different cultures and patterns of social organization. They thus present yet another opportunity for comparison, this time holding constant the political, economic, and physical environment and considering differences in culture.

Hopis have traditionally been sedentary agriculturalists living in villages on or near three mesas in north central Arizona. Navajos have been semisedentary pastoralists occupying a vast area in northwestern New Mexico, northern Arizona, and southern Utah. Their present reservation completely surrounds the Hopi Reservation (see Figure 5-1). We will consider first the histories of how these two peoples came to settle where they are now, their different cultures, and their different patterns of ecological adaptation and social organization and then look at some of the health-related consequences of those differences.

THE HOPI

Hopi is a Shoshonean language that in turn is part of the large family of Uto-Aztecan languages. According to historical linguists, the ancestors of the Hopi entered the Southwest and acquired maize agriculture probably no later than A.D. 500.[2] From the time of their entry into the Southwest until contact with the Spaniards, they have been known from the archaeological record and identified by archaeologists as the Western Anasazi who occupied an area in what is now

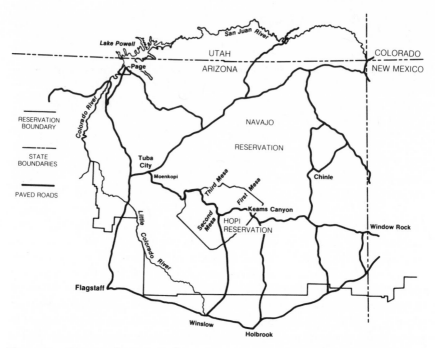

Figure 5-1   Hopi and Navajo Indian reservations, Arizona and Utah, 1970s

northern Arizona and southern Utah that stretched from Chinle Wash in the east to southern Nevada in the west, and from southern Utah as far south as the Little Colorado River. The Western Anasazi remained relatively isolated from other southwestern groups and, before A.D. 1000, were still living in pit-house villages while the Eastern Anasazi of Mesa Verde and the Chaco in northwestern New Mexico already inhabited surface pueblos.[3]

A period of expansion with an increase in population lasted from about 1000 to 1150. There were many small sites, averaging 2.9 rooms and occupied by single extended families. This was a time of improved environmental conditions: Rainfall increased appreciably, and water tables were rising. After 1150, however, the environment began to deteriorate. The people relied more and more on agriculture; their population ceased expanding; and they withdrew from peripheral areas. Some areas were virtually abandoned, and people congregated along lowland drainages and in locations where alluvial farmland and water were available. There developed a discontinuous distribution of sites in which centers of dense population were separated by nearly empty areas. Water tables continued to fall, and erosion increased between 1250 and 1300, when the Western Anasazi relied to an unprecedented degree on agriculture. Gathering diminished in importance as adverse conditions combined to reduce the productivity of natural plant communities. Hunting also contributed less than it had in the preceding period. There was a heightened concern for water. Large sites, concentrated in a few restricted localities, continued trends begun in the previous period. There were, however, few of these, and the majority of settlements continued to be small, located next to arable alluvial bottom land. In some areas there is also evidence of conflict among settlements, presumably because of competition for scarce farmlands.[4]

Beginning about 1300, there was a precipitous drop in the water table, the onset of severe gully cutting, and a significant decrease in rainfall. The entire northern area of the Western Anasazi became unfit for human habitation and people moved to the southern end of Black Mesa, where the Hopi villages are located today, and to a few sites along the Little Colorado River where surface water was still available. By 1450, flooding of the Little Colorado destroyed some villages and irrigation systems, forcing people to join the villages along the southern edge of Black Mesa until only the area occupied by the present-day Hopis was still habitable. These villages were larger and depended on water from springs and seeps at the base of the mesa and from alluvial flooding of the major washes.

Erosion continued until the easternmost Hopi sites, with exception of Awat'ovi, were completely abandoned by the time of the Spanish *entradas*. Spanish estimates of the Hopi population are often unreliable. In 1583, for example, Espejo reported 50,000 Hopis, whereas Luxan said there were 12,000.[5] But estimates of 3,000 in 1614 and 2,966 in 1664 appear more reasonable, if only because they agree with each other and are compatible with the number and size of Hopi sites occupied at the time.

Archaeological evidence has been found of the abandonment of villages due to the erosion of the Jeddito Wash watering the easternmost sites by Antelope Mesa, even after the first Spanish contacts. The archaeological evidence also points to the sporadic occupation of Canyon de Chelly to the east by small groups of Hopis from 1300 to the 19th century but especially before 1700.[6] Ethnographic and historical accounts describe how varying numbers of Hopis were forced to leave their villages during periods of drought and agricultural failure. Spanish sources mention as havens of refuge the Havasupai villages as well as other Pueblos. During the 19th century, Hopis were received at Zuni to the east, and Zunis were hosted at Hopi when their economy was under stress.

In recent years, the view that the 15th- and 16th-century Hopi population was small, that most of the Spanish estimates were exaggerated, and that early ethnographic descriptions reflect the immediate precontact Hopi culture has been contested by those who argue that 14th-century Anasazi society was organized in a complex regional system that collapsed because of organizational failure.[7] This implies a large population, which in turn means that the Spanish estimates of large Hopi populations in the 16th century may well have been more accurate than has generally been supposed. And this means that ethnographic accounts are not a good guide to the social organization of the Pueblos in the precontact period. It also requires an explanation of the much smaller populations estimated in the 18th and 19th centuries. Upham invokes epidemics as the deus ex machina, citing evidence from elsewhere in the New World of depopulation ratios of 20 to 1 or more. Unfortunately there is no evidence of any epidemic in this area at the time, much less a series of epidemics that would selectively eliminate children and young people. Not to worry. Assume a depopulation ratio of 20 to 1 ("an admittedly conservative estimator"[8]); assume not one but two undocumented smallpox epidemics between 1521 and 1581; and presto, a possible scenario becomes a "probable scenario." It should be clear that this revisionist pre- and early contact history is of a piece with the revisionist history of the central place of epidemics in New World depopulation. It is as clear an example as one can find of the assumption of a natural history of population decline among indigenous peoples as a result of European contact.

One of the implications of the revisionist version of western Pueblo prehistory is that despite the absence of large sites before 1400, precontact Hopi society was highly stratified and controlled by an elite.[9] Upham argues that the usual ethnographic view is quite different: that Hopis and other western Pueblos were egalitarian and democratic. This is in fact a highly selective reading of the ethnographic literature, for as Bennett showed almost 50 years ago, there is a deep division between ethnographers who view Hopi society as harmonious, egalitarian, and gemeinschaftlike and those who view it as hierarchical, coercive, and repressive.[10]

Our view is that Hopi society after 1400 was indeed stratified and that it was a system designed to manage scarcity rather than economic surplus.

> The picture that emerges is of a society that maintained stability and integration through the promotion of homogeneity both psychological and structural. Survival depended on unending fieldwork and intense cooperation. To achieve this the ideology had to be egalitarian while all manifestations of individualism—competition, innovation, ambition—were severely discountenanced. At the same time, however, economic reality did not permit equality. The agricultural resources were localized and marginal. During periods of drought, the land could not support the population which had grown during the preceding wet years. A core population had to maintain itself in such a manner that excess population could be sloughed off without creating serious internal conflict. This was achieved by a hierarchical system which concentrated wealth, ceremonial position and status in the hands of a relatively small proportion of families.[11]

Throughout the prehistoric period we see two major developments shaping the evolution of Hopi society: the adoption of agriculture, which most probably led to a transition from bilateral to matrilineal descent, and the effects of the deteriorating environment, which led to population decline and the concentration of a few large villages located by permanent water sources. With the period of abandonment and site aggregation, however, we find the development of the Hopi system as we know it from the ethnographic literature.[12]

Before the adoption of agriculture, Hopi society was very much like that of their linguistic congeners, the Shoshonean speakers of the Great Basin, who occupied an area very similar to that of the Western Anasazi. Subsistence centered around the gathering of wild seeds, roots, and piñon nuts. Extended families came together only occasionally for ceremonies and the piñon harvest. On these occasions, headmen had only temporary authority, there being neither "tribe" nor "band." Women did most of the gathering, and their importance is attested to by matrilocal postnuptial residence, women's control of the seed harvests, and the frequent occurrence of fraternal polyandry in many areas.[13]

Agricultural land in the Southwest is limited so that a rule of inheritance favoring some children at the expense of others evolved in order to avoid dividing fields among heirs to the point that a family could no longer survive. From matrilocal residence and women's control of gathering sites or seed harvests, it is but a step to women's control of farmlands and the inheritance of these lands through the female line.

Early Apachean social organization was very much like that of the Great Basin Shoshoneans except for the agricultural Western Apaches, who developed matrilineal descent. Their settlement pattern was much like that of the Western Anasazi around 1100, that is, many small settlements near farm sites for most of the year. The local group was the largest unit, with a definite leader and important functions. Generally, two or three named clans were represented in each local group, which contained anywhere from two to 10 matrifocal extended families, some containing 10 to 30 households.[14]

In each group, one clan predominated, and the group was known by that clan whether or not it contained others of equal size. The farmlands of a group were spoken of as belonging to its dominant clan, although use rights were not confined to that clan. The head of the local group was also spoken of as the chief of its predominant clan. Marriage to someone of one's own or a related clan was prohibited, but marriage into one's father's clan was preferred, as was the marriage of two people whose fathers were of the same clan (shared father's clan).

If, as we believe is most probable, similar developments took place among the Western Anasazi, a tendency toward local group endogamy would have developed as the reliance on agriculture and group size increased. Successive marriage alliances among two or, at most, three clans sharing localized farm sites decreased internal competition for land. At the same time, however, cultural homogeneity prevailed over fairly large areas, owing to the expanding population and the hiving off of local groups. Relatedness among people of the same clans and phratries (groups of related clans) provided the basis for intersettlement cooperation.

By 1300, when the Hopis abandoned large areas of heretofore habitable land and settled fewer but larger settlements, control of the shrinking agricultural resources led to competition in many locales. The tendency toward local endogamy increased, but the larger village populations contained a greater number of clans, which in turn required the development of mechanisms to integrate the previously autonomous local groups. Marriage prohibitions were developed to preclude the formation of "cliques" resulting from father's clan marriage in successive generations.

With the contraction of the Western Anasazi into the southern Black Mesa area, the social system of the Hopi as we know it today was probably complete. Villages with populations in the hundreds, each containing a large number of clans and phratries, also needed to develop integrative mechanisms beyond that of marriage regulation in order to maintain village harmony, especially during hard times. Presumably, the katsina cult was adopted by the Hopi about this time and was one of the integrating mechanisms. In addition, the power of religious specialists and the emphasis on fertility and rainmaking probably reached their most intense development at this time.

The point to be made by this review of Hopi social history is that there was never a time during which an economic surplus was sufficient to lead to the creation of a managerial class of the sort that, through intervillage marriage alliances, could integrate the numerous villages of both the Western and Eastern Anasazi societies. To the contrary, environmental stress was persistent throughout the entire prehistoric period and not a more recent phenomenon resulting from postcontact conditions. Despite the technological advance represented by agriculture, the health status of the Anasazi Pueblo populations seems to have deteriorated over a long period of time. According to Martin:

> There were major and persistent nutritional deficiencies resulting from a corn diet; crowded and unsanitary living conditions enhanced the chances of picking up communicable diseases such as gastroenteritis; dental problems including caries and periodontal disease were a major concern; most adults had arthritis and spinal degeneration from carrying heavy loads; parasites such as lice and helminths were common; and infant and childhood mortality were high. With respect to trends over time, a continuum of health problems suggests that there were changes in the patterns with an increase in diseases associated with large and aggregated populations.[15]

Among the Hopi, wealth and religious/political power have varied together. Both land and ceremonies are controlled by clans, and the clans with the best lands control the most important ceremonies. Moreover, because ceremonies as well as lands are owned by clans, priestly roles are inherited as a matter of clan membership. Which is to say, Hopi ceremonies are learned by the officiants; they are not a gift that any individual might be born with or acquire as a result of some unusual experience. Finally, as Ruth Underhill observed, because they are agriculturalists, the Hopis direct their ceremonies at bringing rain for the benefit of the entire community rather than for the well-being of a particular individual, as is the case with many of the ceremonies in hunting–gathering societies.[16]

In addition to bringing rain for the benefit of all, public ceremonies may be used as a means of enforcing conformity to community norms. In these densely settled, hierarchically organized villages, mechanisms of social control have been highly developed. Gossip is a powerful, if informal, means. If gossip does not have the desired effect, mocking by clowns at public ceremonies may follow. If all else fails, the leadership of the village may expel deviants. The same institutions that control the religious life of the people also control their behavior, the two spheres often being indistinguishable.

We have said that there is disagreement about the size of the Hopi population before and at contact. There is more general agreement on the size of the population later in the historic period. Mid-19th-century estimates tend to be in the range of 2,500 to 3,000, reaching a nadir after severe drought and the smallpox epidemic of 1866 which reduced the population from around 3,000 to about 1,600 by 1875. Since the turn of the century the population has increased steadily to 2,500 to 3,000 in the 1930s. There was virtually no emigration off the reservation before World War II.[17] After the war, however, emigration increased. In 1980 the U.S. Census enumerated 6,601 Indians on the Hopi Reservation of a total Hopi population of 8,930 (i.e., about 74 percent of the population lived on the reservation).[18] In 1990 the census counted 7,061 Indians on the Hopi Reservation.[19] Despite the difficulties of enumeration and definition, the pattern of population growth over the past 150 years is reasonably clear: stagnation and even decline through the second half of the 19th century followed by a fivefold increase from about 1900 to 1990. As we shall see, the Navajo pattern has been very different.

THE NAVAJOS

Unlike the Hopis, the Navajos appear to be relative newcomers to the Southwest. They are Athabaskan speakers, like other Apacheans, and must have arrived in the Southwest no more than 500 to 700 years ago. They moved into the area at the time the Pueblos had been severely constricted and retrenched. "The Apacheans, including the Eastern Apaches, Western Apaches, and Navajos, located in areas entirely surrounding the Pueblos, and retained intelligibility among the dialects."[20] By 1626, a Spanish report mentioned the Apache Indians of Nabaho, and in 1630, these special Apaches were distinguished from those who never planted but lived by the chase, "whereas the Apaches of Navajo 'are very great farmers.'"[21]

It is generally believed that the Navajos learned farming from the Pueblos and probably developed matrilineal descent at this time. Unlike the clans of the Pueblos, which take their names from animals and natural phenomena, Navajo clan names refer to features of the landscape, much like the band names of the Eastern Apaches. This and the fact that Navajo kinship terminology is not the same as that of any of the Pueblos suggests that matrilineality evolved as an adaptation to their changed subsistence rather than having been borrowed wholesale from the Pueblos.[22] The Navajos also seem to have established fairly sizable villages containing as many as 50 hogans grouped together.[23]

Intensive interaction with the Pueblos began after the Pueblo revolt of 1680 when, in 1690, the Spaniards reconquered the area. From then until about 1770, Tewa, Jemez, Keresan, and Zuni refugees lived among the Navajos. The Navajo population may have doubled at this time, although there is no way of ascertaining its size.[24] The intermixture of populations was such that Hrdlicka observed that contemporary Navajos "are much more closely related both physically and ethnically to the Pueblos" than to the Apaches.[25] The area of Navajo occupation at this time is studded with ruins, called *pueblitos,* containing Pueblo houses intermingled with Navajo hogans. These sites are generally located in defensive locations with walls and lookout towers.[26] It seems likely that this was the period during which the Navajos adopted Pueblo marriage restrictions. Marriage into one's own clan or phratry, one's father's clan and/or phratry, one's shared father's clan and phratry, and one's mother's father's clan and phratry was forbidden, with the result that in a village containing eight or nine exogamous phratries, only about half of the marriageable-age individuals were potential marriage partners.[27] These rules served to integrate the ethnically disparate population by forcing intermarriage. To this fusion the Puebloes brought their knowledge of livestock and religious beliefs, all of which had a profound impact on what was to become "traditional" Navajo culture.

After 1770, drought, intensified Ute raiding, and a resumption of warfare with the Spaniards led to a migration of the Navajos to the south and west of their center of settlement in the upper San Juan River drainage. The relatively large pueblito settlements were abandoned, and the population became more dispersed. Presumably farming diminished somewhat in importance at this time as well, and Pueblo elements of social organization became increasingly more diluted. By the early 1800s, stockraising had become as important as agriculture and, during the early years of the 19th century, became the dominant subsistence pursuit.

Pastoralism led to a dispersed and mobile population. Much of the year was spent in relative isolation in residence groups composed of one extended family from which nuclear families might separate for a variety of reasons and for varying lengths of time. Pastoralism is also, the world over, a male-managed subsistence pursuit associated with patrilocal or virilocal residence and patrilineal descent. Moreover, according to Lowie, the status of women in these societies is "almost uniformly one of decided and absolute inferiority."[28] Yet Navajo society remained matrilineal and has remained so to this day.[29] Low population density and transhumance precluded the development of communitywide ceremonials that marked the Pueblos' agricultural cycle and curing societies. In consequence, Navajo ceremonies are almost exclusively healing rituals performed for individuals. In most other respects, however, the Navajos patterned their religion after that of the Pueblos.

The years from about 1800 to 1863 have been termed the herding and raiding period.[30] The Southwest was ceded by Mexico to the United States in 1848, after which time the federal government sought to control Navajo depredations. In 1864 after an all-out campaign, most of the Navajos were captured and imprisoned at the Bosque Redondo in eastern New Mexico. In 1868 they were allowed to return to a treaty reservation straddling what is now the Arizona–New Mexico border.

After their return from captivity, the Navajos were supplied with livestock and began rebuilding their flocks and herds and spilling over the boundaries of the original Treaty Reservation to return to areas where they had lived previously. Their livestock provided not only subsistence but also wool and meat for sale. The result was increasing integration into the cash economy.

Livestock was not evenly distributed among Navajo family units. As in the period before captivity, so in the later period there were stockmen with large holdings and many dependents to help with the herding, and other families with virtually no stock at all. A survey of the Southern Navajo Reservation in 1915 showed that about a quarter of all families owned no livestock.[31] Even for those with some livestock, pastoralism alone was insufficient to provide complete subsistence, and by the 1920s all but the wealthiest engaged in part-time wage work.[32]

The stock reduction program of the 1930s destroyed the stratification system based on livestock that had evolved before the reservation period and during the first six or seven decades of the reservation period.[33] The result was that virtually no one was able to depend on livestock for subsistence any longer, and the reservation economy shifted to one based on welfare and wage work.

Despite great variations in wealth before stock reduction, Navajo society was never as hierarchical as Hopi society. Navajo positions of leadership were achieved, not inherited. Dependence on a local leader was voluntary. And although various forms of deviant behavior could be sanctioned by the community—including expulsion and death—scattered settlements and the value of personal autonomy meant that there was a great deal of freedom of behavior as well.

Even during the 17th and 18th centuries the Navajo population seems to have been substantial: perhaps 3,000 to 4,000 people, according to various estimates. Over 8,000 were imprisoned in the 1860s, and it is estimated that perhaps another 2,000 remained free, making a total of about 10,000.[34] By 1900, 30 years after their return to their homeland, the population was estimated to be about 20,000. It had doubled by 1930, by which time the reservation had been enlarged to its present size of about 24,000 square miles. By 1960 the population was over 90,000.[35] In 1980 the total Navajo population was said to be 158,633, 104,968 of whom lived on the reservation.[36] According to the 1990 Census, the reservation population was over 143,000. If 66 percent of the total population lived on the reservation, as in 1980, then the total population of Navajos was more than 215,000 in 1990.[37]

There have been major problems counting Indians, including Navajos. Nonetheless, the evidence is persuasive that demographically Navajos have been enormously successful, much more so than any other tribe. Indeed, there is no evidence that they ever suffered the kind of population declines that affected so many other Indian peoples. There are, according to Johnston, "four factors which account for the relative stability of Navaho death rates."

> First, their food supplies were sufficiently stable to permit survival, albeit with much periodic hardship. Secondly, the early cessation of hostilities against the Americans and the effective prohibition of predatory activities both by and against Navahos after 1864 combined to eliminate the heavy male mortality which commonly occurred among Plains Indian tribes. Thirdly, the geographic dispersion of the Navaho effectively insulated them from the worst effects of epidemics which decimated the populations of many densely settled Indian villages and communities. Finally, the profound isolation of most Navahos from outside contacts permitted them to maintain a relatively stable social existence from the time of their return to their homelands in 1869 well into the 20th century.[38]

COMPARATIVE SOCIOECONOMIC PATTERNS

Despite major differences in culture, social organization, settlement patterns, and population history, many of the measures typically associated with health status are strikingly similar among these two tribes. In 1936, as part of the stock reduction program, a major survey of Navajos and Hopis was carried out by the Soil Conservation Service of the Department of Agriculture. Table 5-1 displays some of the summary measures.

Several points stand out. Though the Hopi population was much smaller than the Navajo, their population density was much greater. Consumption groups[39] were larger among Navajos than Hopis. Per capita income was about $10 higher for Hopis than Navajos. The Navajos were, however, more involved in the cash economy than the Hopis were. More of their income was from commercial sources—primarily livestock—and more of their consumption items were pur-

Table 5–1   Population characteristics, Navajo and Hopi Indian reservations, 1936

	Hopi Reservation	Navajo Reservation[a]
Population	2,779	38,360
Population per square mile	3.6	1.5
Average consumption group	5.6	6.8
Income per capita	$149.21	$139.75
Commercial	$ 81.94	$ 97.30
Noncommercial	$ 67.27	$ 42.45
Sources of income	$ 59.53	$ 49.10
Wages	$ 18.19	$ 41.20
Livestock	$ 65.00	$ 32.06
Agriculture	$ 2.22	$ 8.46
Rugs	$ 4.27	$ 8.93
Miscellaneous		
Total stock per capita (sheep units)[b]	11.3	21.0
Total consumption per capita	$108.93	$109.39
Commercial	$ 41.66	$ 66.94
Noncommercial	$ 67.27	$ 42.45
Commercial consumption by kind (in %)		
Food	65	62
Clothing	23	26
Household equipment	7	5
Productive equipment	5	7
Food consumption		
Percent purchased	29	49
Percent home produced	71	51

[a] Figures for the Navajo Reservation also include the Hopi Reservation population, but because there are relatively so few Hopis, the distortion is insignificant.

[b] Sheep units are a unit of measurement for reducing all forms of livestock to a common denominator based on the amount of land required to support one sheep. "A sheep unit is the equivalent of one sheep grazing yearlong. One sheep or goat equals one sheep unit; one head of cattle equals four sheep units; one horse equals five sheep units." The figures are based on the assumption that cattle eat four times as much as sheep do, and horses five times as much. D. F. Aberle, *The Peyote Religion Among the Navajo* (Chicago: Aldine, 1966), p. 67.

Source: Section of Conservation Economics, *Statistical Summary, Human Dependency Survey, Navajo and Hopi Reservations,* Navajo Area, Region 8, Soil Conservation Service (Washington, DC: U.S. Department of Agriculture, 1939).

chased rather than produced by the consumption group. These patterns of income and consumption reflect important differences between the two tribes. Equally important, however, was the fact that their incomes were not dramatically different.

Life changed greatly for both groups within a few years of the Human Dependency Survey. The government-ordered stock reduction had a huge impact on the Navajos,[40] but less on the Hopis, who were not as involved with stock raising. For both tribes World War II and its aftermath brought increasing involvement in wage work, a decline in subsistence agriculture, and a diminution in ceremonial involvement.[41] These changes resulted in rather similar aggregate socioeconomic measures, as Table 5-2 indicates.

There is some evidence that the Hopis have participated more fully in the educational system, a point to which we shall return later. Apart from that, measures of poverty, labor force participation, and unemployment are remarkably similar. Moreover, both reservations occupy similar peripheral positions in the national economy. In each case, whatever natural resources exist are extracted by non-Indian interests, with relatively few benefits flowing to reservation residents in the form of jobs. Indeed, most wage employment is in the health, education, and welfare bureaucracies of government agencies. In regard to socioeconomic measures, therefore, the two populations have been remarkably similar for at least 50 years.

Regarding access to health care, too, the Navajos and Hopis are similar. Since

Table 5–2 Socioeconomic measures, Navajo and Hopi reservations, 1970 and 1980

	Hopi Reservation		Navajo Reservation	
	1970	1980	1970	1980
Proportion of housing with >1 person/room	65.8	58.0	75.8	64.9
Proportion of units <10 years old	9.2	33.1	54.0	47.1
Proportion of people ≥25 years old who are high school graduates	27.5	40.3	17.4	34.6
Proportion of people ≥16 years old in the labor force	36.4	54.7	32.9	58.3
Unemployment rate	13.7	20.5	12.0	23.7
Proportion of traditional occupations	—	6.3	—	4.5
Median family income	$6,839	8,197	6,106	8,397
Proportion of families below poverty	61.8	50.9	62.1	50.5
Proportion who have always lived on the reservation	—	91.2	—	89.7

Source: C. M. Snipp, *American Indians: The First of this Land* (New York: Russell Sage Foundation, 1989), various pages. Data from 1970 and 1980 are not comparable, owing to boundary changes.

1955 Indian residents of each reservation have been beneficiaries of the Indian Health Service and have received free medical care as well as a variety of community health services. Before 1955 these services were provided by the Bureau of Indian Affairs. Similarly, access to social services from the Bureau of Indian Affairs and from state and county governments are essentially the same. Thus both reservations are strikingly similar to the MIRAB economies described in Chapter 3. Possibilities for economic growth have not been realized; wage work is found primarily off the reservation or in government agencies on the reservation; and those who cannot find adequate employment are dependent on welfare and a variety of subsistence activities.

DIFFERENCES IN HEALTH

Population Change

We have shown that the Navajo population has grown to a much greater size than has the Hopi population. Over the past century the number of Hopis has increased perhaps fivefold (from 1,900 to 9,000), whereas the number of Navajos has increased more than 10-fold (from 20,000 to >200,000). There also is evidence of more rapid Navajo than Hopi growth in the 19th century: from 1800 to the 1860s perhaps threefold for the former, as contrasted with no growth for the latter.

Observers during the early years of this century commented on the differences in the health of the Navajos and Hopis. The Hopis were said to live in less sanitary conditions than the Navajos and to experience worse health and higher infant death rates.[42] Several epidemics of smallpox afflicted the Hopis in the second half of the 19th century (1853, 1866, and 1899), whereas there is no record of such events among the Navajos.[43] As noted in Chapter 1, a sequence of epidemics such as this is especially likely to cause the population to fall, as the youngest generation is afflicted preferentially after the first epidemic.

Less impressionistically, an analysis of the 1900 census showed that among Hopi women aged 18 to 52, the average number of children ever born was 5.7, with an average of 2.9 still alive. In contrast, among Navajos the corresponding figures were 4.4 ever born and 3.6 still alive.[44] Thus in the late 19th century, Hopi fertility was higher and child survival was lower than they were among the Navajos, thus indicating that infertility and subfertility have not always been implicated in population decline, as some writers have suggested.[45]

There were also measurable differences in the fertility and population profiles of the villages of First and Second Mesas, which suffered more from the epidemics than did Orayve on Third Mesa. Thirty-eight percent of the Navajos in the area and 34 percent of the Orayves were between 0 and 9 years of age, compared to 21 percent for the villages of First and Second Mesa.[46] In general, Orayve's population was much younger than the populations of First and Second Mesas (see Table 5-3). In addition, there were significant differences in the number of childless women over 33 years of age, their fertility rates, and the proportion

Table 5–3 Intermesa comparisons of age cohorts

A. Adults and children

| | Mesa | | | | | | |
| | First | | Second | | Third | | |
Age	Obs	(Exp)	Obs	(Exp)	Obs	(Exp)	Total
≥20	301	(286.57)	319	(286.57)	411	(457.87)	1,031
≤19	236	(250.43)	218	(250.43)	447	(400.13)	901
	537		537		858		1,932

Note: $X^2 = 19.75$; *df* = 2; *p* = .0001.

B. Adults 20+ years of age

| | Mesa | | | | | | |
| | First | | Second | | Third | | |
Age	Obs	(Exp)	Obs	(Exp)	Obs	(Exp)	Total
40+	137	(128.46)	177	(136.14)	126	(175.4)	440
30–39	91	(84.08)	68	(89.11)	129	(114.81)	288
20–29	73	(88.46)	74	(93.75)	156	(120.79)	303
	301		319		411		1,031

Note: $X^2 = 51.19$; *df* = 4; *p* = <.0001.

Source: J. E. Levy, *Orayve Revisited: Social Stratification in an "Egalitarian" Society* (Santa Fe: School of American Research, 1992).

of surviving children (see Table 5-4).[47] According to Bradfield, the epidemic of 1853 hit the First Mesa villages the hardest, and that of 1866/67 was worst for the villages of the Second Mesa.[48] The government successfully quarantined Orayve during the epidemic of 1899, with the result that the village was spared and its population in 1900 looked more like that of the Navajos than did those of the other mesas.

Anthropologists working in Hopi villages starting in the 1930s also commented on the differences between the Navajos and Hopis. Colton noted that the Navajos moved seasonally, that their water supplies were uncontaminated because they were far from dwellings, and that the excreta deposited "not far" from their dwellings "do not present a menace to health because of the sparsity of the population and the semiarid climate."[49] He continued: "The Hopi family, on the other hand, lives in crowded quarters. Families live close together, and the excreta are often deposited in the narrow plazas, streets, middens, and passages near the houses. Were it not for the arid climate, living conditions would be impossible."[50]

Writing in the 1950s about his early fieldwork at the Third Mesa village of Orayve, Titiev observed:

Toilet habits have changed markedly. In the 1930s young boys, in particular, did not hesitate to urinate on the terraces before their houses. They were warned only not to wet and thus weaken the walls. At present they go to the edge of the mesa to relieve

Table 5–4 Fertility and survival of children on three mesas (women 33+ years of age)

A. Fertility (as # children born/fertile woman) and survival rates of children

Mesa[a]	Barren	Bearing	Total	Fertility	% Surviving
First Mesa	9	71	80	6.51	40.7
Second Mesa	8	82	90	7.34	35.2
Third Mesa	3	80	83	8.09	47.5
Navajo[b]	2	129	131	5.3	79.4

B. Survival of children

Mesa	Died		Survived		Total
	Obs	Exp	Obs	Exp	
First	274	(271.1)	188	(190.9)	462
Second	390	(353.2)	212	(248.75)	602
Third	340	(379.7)	307	(267.3)	647
	1004		707		1711

Note: $X^2 = 19.4$; $df = 2$; $p = <.0001$.

[a]*Source:* J. E. Levy, *Orayve Revisited: Social Stratification in an "Egalitarian" Society* (Sanfe Fe: School of American Research, 1992).

[b]*Source:* S. R. Johansson and S. H. Preston, "Tribal demography: The Hopi and Navajo populations as seen through manuscripts from the 1900 U.S. Census," *Social Science History* 3 (1978):1–33.

themselves, and house terraces no longer reek of stale urine. As for defecation, members of both sexes used to resort to the outskirts of the pueblo and trusted to cultural blindness to preserve their modesty. These conditions no longer prevail.[51]

Different living conditions accounted for the differences in mortality from both epidemic and endemic infectious diseases. The fertility differences documented from the 1900 census cannot be accounted for as readily. It has generally been said that contraception was not widely used by either group.[52] On the other hand, an army surgeon at the Bosque Redondo in the 1860s is quoted in reference to the Navajos:

On this reservation I cannot say I have seen a single case of constitutional syphilis. But what does and will decrease the number of the tribe and finally wipe them out of existence is the extensive system of abortion carried on by the young women. You may remark how seldom it is a young woman has a child; in fact, none of the women, except they are thirty or forty, ever think of having one, if they can help it, so that two or three children are considered a large family.[53]

Admittedly this was an especially traumatic period of Navajo history, and women may have been especially likely to have wanted to avoid having children in such a setting. Nonetheless, it is also possible that such voluntary restriction continued to be practiced, particularly among women who were over 30 at the time of the 1900 census and who were of the generation born at the Bosque Redondo or in the years preceding captivity.

It is also possible that the pastoralists walking long distances each day–as many Navajo women did when herding sheep—might be less fecund than women in agricultural communities. Research elsewhere suggests that sedentism is associated with greater fecundity than is hunting-gathering. The same may be true of pastoralism. Without knowing more about the daily activities of women at the time, however, we can do no more than speculate. The reasons for the low Navajo fertility in the late 19th century therefore still eludes us. We can say, however, that before medical treatment and public health had much to offer American Indians, patterns of child mortality and fertility varied in ways that were associated with the ecological adaptations that each had made. The fertility differences do not accord with the high levels of sterility suggested as being among the major determinants of population decline, for the population that was declining had a higher fertility rate than the one that was increasing.

Cultural factors also appear to have had an effect on both the children's survival and the fertility of women in Orayve, the one village not affected by the epidemic of 1899. Although there were no significant differences in the average number of children born to women between the ages of 18 and 32, after age 33 women of the senior lineages in high-ranking clans had significantly *more* children per bearing woman than did all other women. These women of the highest possible status not only bore more children (10 per woman over 33 years as compared with 7.5 for all other women in the same age cohort), but their children also had the poorest survival rates (28.6 versus 47.3 percent). It would appear that rather than controlling birthrates, the high-status women were trying to produce heirs and so tended to shorten birth spacing, thus displacing the older sibling from the breast and inadvertently exposing it to a variety of infectious diseases. In an effort to preserve their positions, the senior lineages of the leading clans, it seems, were engaging in a self-defeating practice.[54]

Fertility in the Postwar Era

By the early 1970s there had been a striking reversal in the fertility rates of Navajos and Hopis. The former had an average annual crude rate in 1971/72 of between 28 and 34 per 1,000, depending on the population estimate. The latter had a rate of between 18.9 and 20.8 per 1,000 population (on the reservation).[55] Moreover, it was clear that the reason the Hopi birthrate was lower than the Navajos' was that the Hopis had significantly lower numbers of births at ages 30 and above. Hopis in their 30s and above had higher rates of induced abortions, hysterectomies, and bilateral tubal ligations than did Navajos of the same age.[56] Vasectomies were equally uncommon in each population.

There are no data available on the use of oral contraceptives and IUDs among Hopis. Data from the Navajo population indicate that IUD use was as effective as in most populations but that oral contraceptives were used less effectively than in any other populations studied at the time.[57] Ineffectiveness was due to "personal" rather than "medical" reasons, usually the objections of husbands, boyfriends, and family members.[58]

Interviews with Navajo women indicated that those who were likely to use contraception were older, had more than three children, had less than an eighth-grade education, and lived in arrangements in which they were relatively less dependent on kin than were the nonusers. The interviews suggested that most of the women with many children were interested in knowing how to control their fertility but that pressure from their mothers and husbands discouraged it. Those who lived relatively independent of kin thus avoided many of those pressures. On the other hand, young women were not particularly likely to be contraceptive users.[59] These data suggest part of the reason that Navajo fertility rates remained high into the 30s and 40s. They do not indicate why the Hopi rates did not. To explain that we must turn to other sources.

One of the variables often observed to be associated with declining fertility is female education. In 1970, 52 percent of Hopi women 25 to 34 years of age had graduated from high school, compared with 28.8 percent of Navajo women of that age.[60] For men the figures were 58.3 and 35.5 percent. Thus, although the educational differences between the two tribes were not enormous when all people 25 and above were included (see Table 5-2), among young adults the differences were substantial, suggesting that the postwar changes had had a greater impact on the Hopis than on the Navajos.

Much of the difference can be explained by differences in settlement patterns. Hopis live in compact villages; Navajos live in more or less isolated camps. The construction of a paved road in the late 1950s linking all the Hopi villages to one another and to off-reservation towns had profound consequences because the Hopis now had easy access to the high school built on the reservation in the 1930s as well as to sources of entertainment, shopping, and employment in non-Indian communities.[61] Titiev wrote of the changes brought about in the village of Orayve by the new road network:

> The inhabitants no longer feel isolated, and no longer are they impelled to direct their energies inward toward the village and to develop internal strength through self-reliance, pueblo-wide ceremonies, local amusements, and communal enterprises. Instead, people now turn their attention outward and away from the pueblo, especially in such matters as jobs, shopping, and entertainment.[62]

Because we do not have interview data, we may infer only tentatively that it was changes such as those described by Titiev that were involved in the dramatic decline of fertility among women aged 30 and above.

Increasing educational levels and diminished isolation of the villages were also implicated in a decline in the ceremonial cycle, in a shift from a primarily subsistence to a primarily cash economy, in the use of modern construction techniques and materials that enabled the building of new and larger homes, and in the tendency for nuclear families to reside independently.[63] A scattered population and larger numbers meant that many of these same changes have taken much longer to be felt in Navajo society. Indeed, only in the last decade has urbanization become the dominant mode for most Navajos.

Morbidity and Mortality

The postwar years saw an impressive decline in the death rates in each population, so much so that by the 1960s noninfectious and man-made conditions had come to dominate the epidemiologic regimes of each population. Infant mortality had dropped dramatically in each tribe: For the Hopis in 1968/69 the rate was 11.4 per 1,000 live births, and the Navajos in 1970 had a rate of 31.5, a substantial decline since the prewar years.[64] Accidents of all sorts were the leading cause of death in each population. Motor vehicle accidents accounted for about half of all accidents in each, and in the mid-1970s the Hopi rate was at least half the Navajo rate.

Comparisons of mortality pattern using officially reported statistics are made difficult, however, by the way they are aggregated. Navajo deaths are reported for the "Navajo Area," which comprises not only the reservation itself but also the nearby towns of Flagstaff, Winslow, and Holbrook, Arizona, and Gallup and Farmington, New Mexico, and some more sparsely settled regions. Any Indian who dies in these places is counted as a Navajo, even though Indians of other tribes also live there. For the Hopis, on the other hand, deaths are reported for the Indian Health Service catchment area (service unit) which comprises the Hopi reservation.

Because the number of Navajos in the region is so large compared with other Indian populations, this reporting convention does not distort their mortality patterns to an intolerable degree. But it can have a substantial impact on the patterns reported for much smaller tribes if, as is assuredly the case, there is selection at work. For instance, if Hopis who migrate to border towns are more likely than Hopis who remain on reservation to have drinking problems, then when they die of alcohol-related conditions, their deaths will be counted with the Navajo figures and not with the Hopis'. To circumvent this problem, we describe only conditions on which actual field studies have been carried out. We shall discuss the comparative epidemiology of two chronic conditions in order to make the point that even after major cultural and socioeconomic changes are well under way and even when access to health care is free and essentially available on demand, there still are major differences in behavior in the two tribes that are reflected in differences in patterns of disease.

Alcoholic Cirrhosis

Alcohol has widely been regarded as the most destructive of the trade items that Europeans provided to the indigenous peoples of the New World and Oceania. Most commonly the effects of excessive consumption have been judged by the public behavior that is readily observable: public intoxication, group drinking, brawling, motor vehicle accidents, and so on. Another way to measure the effects is to use the incidence of death due to, or the prevalence of, alcoholic cirrhosis. This condition is the result of heavy, prolonged drinking that may or may not also involve the more public behaviors just cited.

Because Navajos have commonly used alcohol in public and usually in groups, it has been the conventional wisdom for decades that alcohol is their "number one health problem," to quote a commonly used phrase. On the other hand, because the Hopis have presented themselves, and have been perceived by many others, as the peaceful people living in harmonious and well-integrated communities, alcohol abuse has not been widely remarked on until relatively recently.

As a result, it came as a surprise when we observed in the 1960s that the Hopi death rate from alcoholic cirrhosis was over 40 per 100,000, more than twice the Navajo rate, which was no more than 17.3 per 100,000. So surprising was it, indeed, that one senior clinician in the Indian Health Service (IHS) accused us of falsifying the data, despite the fact that all the cases were diagnosed in IHS hospitals, some on the very service for which he was responsible. Because the Hopi population is not numerous—in those years numbering between 5,000 and 6,000—one or two deaths a year would not strike most observers as unusual. It was only by calculating the rate of death that we became aware that alcohol abuse was a problem. Moreover, of the eight Hopis who died of cirrhosis in the years 1965–67, only one had been living on the reservation at the time of death. The others lived off the reservation in border towns and would have been counted as Navajo deaths in the official statistics.

Originally we assumed that the reason that most of these deaths had occurred off the reservation was that people had been unable to resist the temptations of easy access to alcohol in the towns and that town life itself had been so stressful and disruptive that they had turned to alcohol for relief. The picture was more complex, however, for the survivors of the people who had died, as well as families of other cirrhotics we interviewed, often said that the drinking had begun on the reservation and that the family had been pressured to leave the community when social sanctions had been unable to change the drinker's behavior. Not every community was able to exert pressure on the deviants to leave, however. For as we and others have observed, in some villages where the existing ceremonial cycle and theocratic structure had ceased to operate, such mechanisms of social control could no longer be invoked.[65]

The most salient distinction between villages at the time of our study was whether or not they had accepted the legitimacy of the federally instituted tribal council. The anticouncil villages were those where the theocracy still excercised influence and thus where traditional mechanisms of social control could still be enforced. Such mechanisms included as a last resort the expulsion of deviants from the community. In the procouncil villages such mechanisms were no longer intact, and deviants could not be expelled. Thus when we compared all cirrhotics —not simply those who had died—by current residence, we found significantly more living off than on the reservation and more in procouncil than in anticouncil villages. But when we compared them by village of origin, there was no difference between anticouncil and procouncil villages.[66]

The next question was how to explain the origin of deviant behavior within the villages. In this instance there were not enough cases of alcoholic cirrhosis to analyze, and we therefore analyzed together several extreme deviant acts, including homicide, suicide, and all forms of alcohol-related pathology.

We have already said that Hopi villages were endogamous and that a variety of marriage rules precluded the formation of political cliques through marriage alliances. We observed in the procouncil villages that the social deviants were more likely than the controls were to be the products of disapproved intermesa marriages or marriages with non-Hopis. This, however, was not the case in the anticouncil villages where all marriages in the parent generation adhered to the rule of village or mesa endogamy. On the other hand, the social deviants in the anticouncil villages were more likely than the controls were to be the offspring of marriages of people from clans of very different statuses.[67]

Thus it appears that deviant behavior of several types, including alcohol abuse, has been more likely in the children of disapproved marriages and that such disapproved marriages could and did occur within the traditional system as well as the nontraditional system. Indeed, in the traditional system, marriage between members of clans of different status was common, considering both the small size of Hopi villages in past times and the further limitation placed by the numerous marriage proscriptions on the number of suitable partners available. In the nontraditional system in the anticouncil villages in the mid-1960s, clan status was not significant, as control of land and ceremonies had diminished in importance. On the other hand, the parents' village of origin still seemed to be important. It is unlikely that clan, village, or mesa remains as salient to the present generation of young adult Hopis as they were even a generation ago.

The Navajo situation was different. There are reports from at least the late 19th century that the use of alcohol was common among Navajos, particularly men. Men would drink with others of the same age, often at ceremonies and generally with relatives and friends. Alcohol was expensive and an item of high prestige, and thus another common form of consumption was for a wealthy stockman to give it to the dependent members of his outfit. In such situations it was not uncommon for the women also to have a drink.[68] In all these instances, alcohol use was a social activity. Indeed, the person who drank alone and did not share his alcohol was considered to be deviant. Moreover, the Navajos have not cherished the value of self-restraint to quite the same degree as have the Hopis and other Western Pueblos. Thus flamboyant drinking behavior among groups of young men particularly has not been discountenanced as it has among Hopis.

In this context, heavy drinking among groups of men was not considered deviant, and most men who lived in remote areas and who drank in this way went for weeks or months without drinking at all. Moreover, because such behavior was so widely accepted and promoted group solidarity, family members were unable or unwilling to intervene even if excessive drinking had untoward consequences, as it often did, for accidents, fights, arrests, and the expenditure of needed cash were not uncommon. Alcoholic cirrhosis was not high on the list of consequences, however, because the style of drinking coupled with the isolation of so many Navajo families made steady drinking unlikely.[69] In the next chapter we shall consider some of the differences between people who died of cirrhosis and other consequences of alcohol abuse and those who used alcohol a lot but did not die of the consequences. Suffice it to say here that most men substantially reduced their alcohol consumption as they entered their 40s. Those who did not were a minority.

Not only was the mortality rate from cirrhosis higher among Hopis than Navajos, but the evidence also suggested that the case-fatality rate (the proportion of people with the disease who died of it) was higher as well. That is, once someone had developed cirrhosis, death occurred in a higher proportion of cases, indicating that the disease had a different natural history in each population. It is clear, therefore, that the incidence and trajectory of cirrhosis were different in these two neighboring Indian populations; which is to say, the natural history of the condition differed in ways related to the social organization and culture of each tribe.

Epilepsy

Epilepsy is a chronic condition caused by a number of different phenomena, including infection, trauma, and alcohol abuse. Much of the time the cause is unknown (idiopathic epilepsy). It is somewhat more prevalent among Indian than Anglo-American populations but less prevalent than in poverty-stricken areas, especially inner cities. In a study of epilepsy among Navajos and several Pueblo tribes, Levy and colleagues found that in comparison with the prevalence among whites in Rochester, Minnesota (5.7 per 1,000), the age-adjusted rates among Indians were as follows: Tewas, 7.5; Navajos, 8.2; Hopis, 8.0; and Zunis, 9.1.

Seventy-five percent of the Anglo-American cases were idiopathic, whereas 47 percent of the Indian cases were. The higher prevalence of epilepsy among Indians, and the relatively lower proportion of idiopathic cases, was explained by the greater exposure of Indians to infection, trauma, and excessive alcohol consumption.[71] For our purposes, what is important is the trajectory of epilepsy among Navajos and Pueblos (including Hopis). Navajo epileptics were significantly more likely than Pueblos were to have developed emotional and social problems. Among epileptics with such problems, Navajos developed them earlier. And among people with problems, female, but not male, Navajo epileptics developed far more severe problems than did Pueblo epileptics.

> Only Navajos (two males and one female) were diagnosed as psychotic. Only Navajos were involved in homicide or homicide attempts: two females were murdered, one male was murdered by his brother, and another was seriously stabbed by his brother. Only Navajos (two males and one female) made serious suicide attempts. Seven Navajo women were diagnosed as having persistent hysterical reactions and another had a few isolated episodes. One Pueblo male also had a few episodes.[72]

Levy and associates attribute the earlier onset and greater severity of emotional and social problems among Navajo epileptics to differences in the ways in which parents respond to children with a seizure disorder. "The characteristic reaction of Navajo parents to the epileptic child was withdrawal," even to the extent of fleeing when a child had a seizure. "By contrast, Pueblo parents tried to treat the epileptic child as normally as possible. They took special pains to talk with their own and their neighbors' children, so that they would act calmly when witnessing a convulsion and would not tease." However, "the outward placidity of Pueblo parents masked a tendency to deny the serious and chronic nature of the disease. . . . By treating the child as normal, Pueblo parents avoided dealing with the medical and social problems posed by the disease." The result was that when Pueblo children with epilepsy entered adolescence, they tended to develop emotional problems, just as the Navajo children did, though not of the same severity.[73]

Why do Navajos and Pueblos deal with epileptics so differently? Levy and colleagues argue that Navajos view epilepsy as the result of incest, whereas Hopis and other Pueblos do not. Why, then, is incest of so much greater concern to Navajos than to Hopis and other Pueblo Indians?

The admittedly speculative explanation is that when the Athabaskans moved into the Southwest some time before the Spanish *entrada,* they had bilateral descent and practiced cross-cousin marriage, which was later to become a preference for marriage into the father's clan after the development of matrilineal descent. We have seen that as a result of hosting many Pueblos for almost a century after the Spanish reconquest in the 1690s, the Navajos adopted Pueblo marriage proscriptions so as to integrate polities composed of different cultures (Pueblos and Athabaskans). Later, when pastoralism became the dominant pursuit and the population dispersed, families lived in relative isolation for much of the year. A taboo that once had threatened punishment for not marrying into different ethnic groups changed and came to refer only to marriage within one's own clan. Violation of the prohibition was believed to cause epilepsy.[74] Where social controls were largely lacking, supernatural sanctions were more likely to be invoked.

That is to say, clan incest became a major preoccupation for the Navajos because they resided in isolated family units where incest was a real risk. Among Pueblos residing in densely settled villages where public scrutiny was continuous, incest was less likely. Thus the meaning of epilepsy was especially charged for the Navajos, whereas it was not for the Pueblos, and thus the familial and societal reaction to epilepsy was different as well, with different consequences for the epileptic.

DISCUSSION

The Navajos and the Hopis have been in contact for about 500 years and have profoundly influenced each other. Nonetheless they remain quite distinct. That this continues to be the case is attributable to the fact that for Indians it was land that the encroaching European-Americans wanted, and it was acquired by means of both warfare and treaties. The treaties recognized Indian tribes as domestic sovereign nations with legitimate claims to certain territories and certain rights. The situation was different from that of, for example, African Americans, from whom labor rather than land was the desired commodity. For Africans, tribal distinctions were vaporized in the crucible of slavery and its aftermath. The result was the establishment of an African-American identity that long antedates the creation, however incomplete, of a supratribal, American Indian identity. It was indeed the establishment of reservations recognized by treaty that has made possible the continual reaffirmation of tribal, as distinguished from a more generalized Indian, identity.[75]

Even before the reservation period, the histories of population change were different in each tribe. In the early reservation years before medical interventions were very effective, they continued to be different. The reasons for these different population trajectories have nothing to do with widespread infertility among Hopis, a cause of population decline that has been invoked in Polynesia and that has been suggested as a model for the American Indian decline. Whatever the causes elsewhere, among the Hopis there is no evidence of infertility, suggesting that it is possible to reach the same point by several paths. Moreover, among the Navajos, population growth in the late 19th century was associated with comparatively low fertility, but with even lower mortality.

Among the Indians north of Mexico the Navajos are unique, for there is no evidence that they ever suffered the declines experienced by so many other native Americans, even in the 16th century when, it is postulated, a smallpox pandemic decimated the Indians even before they saw their first European.[76] We have already suggested some of the reasons: a scattered settlement pattern, relative isolation, a reservation that was expanded by executive order several times until the 1930s, and encouragement to be independent by agents of the federal government, who in the early reservation period provided livestock so that herds and flocks could be rebuilt. Like the several Polynesian populations described in Chapter 3, the Navajos are important because they exemplify the fact that disease did not afflict all populations in the same fashion or to the same degree and that to invoke disease as the cause of the universal decline of New World populations in the absence of other factors is to oversimplify. Indeed, it seems implausible that Navajos alone should have escaped unscathed while every other population declined by 90 percent or so. More plausible is a whole spectrum of responses, from the Navajos at one end to total extinction at the other.[77]

In the contemporary era, too, we have shown that diversity continues to characterize fertility, mortality and the consequences of chronic disease. As in the case of epidemics of acute infectious diseases, so in the case of noninfectious chronic conditions, diseases do not simply happen to a society; they are as well an expression of that society. The comparisons between Navajo and Hopi cirrhotics and epileptics illustrate an alternative way of conceiving of disease trajectories: as careers of people with a particular condition in contrast with the natural history of the condition itself. In an essay on longitudinal studies of alcohol abuse, Griffith Edwards called attention to these two different models used by investigators to explain the patterns they observed. He defined natural history as "the sequential development of designated biological processes within the individual" and career "as an individual's sequential behaviour within a designated role."[78]

There is an important epistemological difference between the conceptions of natural history and career. We have already said that the former assumes a natural world free of adventitious human influences. It is essentialist in its view of disease. Which is to say, it is assumed that diseases may be treated as species with an existence and course largely independent of the characteristics of the individuals or populations who suffer from them. Those who write about patient (or deviant) careers tend to take a more nominalist view. They do not necessarily deny the reality of harmful biological processes but argue that they do not exist as diseases until they have been defined as diseases. And what is crucial, the very process of defining or labeling a condition as a disease rather than, say, a sin has profound implications for the person experiencing the condition and for the outcome of the condition.[79]

Writers who use the idea of career to describe the experiences of patients are concerned with how the patient's sense of self is shaped by the institutions and individuals with which his condition brings him in contact. According to Erving Goffman,

> One value of the concept of career is its two-sidedness. One side is linked to internal matters held dearly and closely, such as image of self and felt identity; the other side concerns official positions, jural relations, and style of life, and is part of a publicly accessible institutional complex. The concept of career, then, allows one to move back and forth between the personal and the public, between the self and its significant society.[80]

A number of studies of patients with particular conditions have been based on this notion of career, among them Goffman's work with mental patients. Julius Roth's[81] with tuberculosis patients, Fred Davis's[82] with polio patients, and Robert Scott's[83] with blind people. The study of the blind suggests that people with the same level of disability may be taught to be independent or dependent, according to the treatment philosophy of the program providing services. Likewise, the differences between Hopi and Navajo epileptics and cirrhotics may best be viewed as differences in the typical careers of people with these conditions in each culture, rather than as differences in the natural history of the two conditions.

All these examples are based on chronic conditions that are slowly, or not inevitably, fatal and in which what people are taught to believe about themselves makes a difference in regard to their outcome. These contrast with conditions such as lung cancer, which are equally fatal regardless of therapy or socioeconomic status.[84] In such conditions it makes more sense to talk about the natural history of the disease than the career of the patient, at least in regard to outcome. The career conception is thus particularly useful in explaining the course of conditions in which the patient's own behavior may have a determining influence on outcome, because it speaks to the way in which social institutions shape how people conceive of themselves and how conceptions of the self shape the course of the condition.[85]

The contrasting historical and contemporary experiences of these two neighboring peoples therefore indicate that in regard to both acute infectious diseases and chronic diseases, the conception of "natural history of disease" may be misleading. The epidemiology of acute infectious diseases, whether epidemic or endemic, and chronic diseases, whether infectious (tuberculosis) or noninfectious (epilepsy) all are shaped in important but different ways by the social context in which they occur. It is only by understanding this context that one can understand morbidity and mortality in their full complexity.

NOTES

1. S. Nagata, *Modern Transformations of Moenkopi Pueblo* (Urbana: University of Illinois Press, 1970); S. Nagata, "The reservation community and the urban community," in J. O. Waddell and O. M. Watson, eds., *The American Indian in Urban Society* (Boston: Little, Brown, 1971), pp. 114–59; R. O. Clemmer, *Continuities of Hopi Culture Change* (Ramona, CA: Acoma Books, 1978); D. F. Aberle, "A plan for Navajo economic development," in *Toward Economic Development for Native American Communities,* a compendium of papers submitted to the Sub-Committee on Economy in Government of the Joint Economic Committee of the Congress of the United States (Washington, DC: U.S. Government Printing Office, 1969); J. E. Levy, "Who benefits from energy resource development: The special case of the Navajo Indians," *Social Science Journal* 17(1980): 1–19.

2. J. G. Jorgensen, *Western Indians: Comparative Environments, Languages, and Cultures of 172 Western American Indian Tribes* (San Francisco: Freeman, 1980), p. 68.

3. G. G. Gumerman and J. S. Dean, "Prehistoric cooperation and competition in the Western Anasazi area," in L. S. Cordell and G. G. Gumerman, eds., *Dynamics of Southwest Prehistory* (Washington, DC: Smithsonian Institution Press (a School of American Research Advanced Seminar Book), 1989), pp. 99–148, 111.

4. J. Haas and W. Creamer, "Warfare and tribalization in the prehistoric Southwest: Report on the first season's work, 1984" (Santa Fe: School of American Research Press, 1985).

5. E. G. McIntire, "Hopi Indian population change," paper presented at the 14th annual meeting of the Arizona Academy of Science, Phoenix, April 18, 1970; E. H. Spicer, *Cycles of Conquest: The Impact of Spain, Mexico, and the United States on the Indians of the Southwest, 1533–1960* (Tucson: University of Arizona Press, 1962), p. 190.

6. C. R. Steen, *Tse Ta'a: Excavations at Tse Ta'a, Canyon de Chelly National Monument, Arizona,* Research Series no. 9 (Washington, DC: National Park Service, 1966), pp. 55–57.

7. S. Upham, *Politics and Power: An Economic and Political History of the Western Pueblo* (New York: Academic Press, 1982).

8. S. Upham, "Smallpox and climate in the American Southwest," *American Anthropologist* 88(1986):126.

9. It may be more accurate to put the sequence the other way around. Size and complexity are assumed, and a mechanism must be discovered or invented to account for the fact that what Europeans described was smaller and, in some instances, simpler.

10. J. Bennett, "The interpretation of Pueblo culture: A question of values," *Southwestern Journal of Anthropology* 2(1946):361–74. See also R. Redfield, *The Little Community: Viewpoints for a Study of a Human Whole* (Chicago: University of Chicago Press, 1955).

11. J. E. Levy, S. J. Kunitz, and E. B. Henderson, "Hopi deviance in historical and epidemiological perspective," in L. Donald, ed., *Themes in Ethnology and Culture History: Essays in Honor of David F. Aberle* (Berkeley, CA: Folklore Institute, 1987), p. 385.

12. For a more detailed discussion of Hopi society and population, see J. E. Levy,

Orayve Revisited: Social Stratification in an "Egalitarian" Society (Santa Fe: School of American Research Press, 1992).

13. F. Eggan, "Shoshone Kinship Structures and Their Significance for Anthropological Theory," *Journal of the Steward Anthropological Society* 11(1980):65–93.

14. R. N. Bellah, *Apache Kinship Systems* (Cambridge, MA: Harvard University Press, 1952); G. Goodwin, *The Social Organization of the Western Apache* (1st ed. 1942) (Tucson: University of Arizona Press, 1969).

15. D. L. Martin, "Patterns of health and disease: Stress profiles for the prehistoric Southwest," paper prepared for The Organization and Evolution of Prehistoric Southwestern Society, advanced seminar, School of American Research, Santa Fe, September 25–29, 1989.

16. R. Underhill, *Ceremonial Patterns in the Greater Southwest*, American Ethnological Society, Monograph no. 13 (Seattle: University of Washington Press, 1948), p. viii.

17. E. G. McIntire, "Hopi Indian population change," paper presented at the 14th annual meeting of the Arizona Academy of Science, Phoenix, April 18, 1970, on file in the library of the Museum of Northern Arizona, Flagstaff.

18. C. M. Snipp, *American Indians: The First of this Land* (New York: Russell Sage Foundation 1989), pp. 87, 328ff.

19. E. Palsano, J. Greendeer-Lee, J. Cowles, and D. Carroll, *American Indian and Alaska Native Areas, 1990* (Washington, DC: Racial Statistics Branch, Population Division, Bureau of the Census, 1991).

20. Jorgensen, *Western Indians,* pp. 71–72.

21. R. M. Underhill, *The Navajos* (Norman: University of Oklahoma Press, 1956), pp. 35–36.

22. Although the prevailing opinion is that the Navajos and Western Apaches developed matrilineal descent after their arrival in the Southwest, Dyen and Aberle attempted to demonstrate that the Apacheans were matrilineal before they left their northern homeland in what is now Alaska and western Canada and that the Eastern Apaches became bilateral after their arrival. See I. Dyen and D. F. Aberle, *Lexical Reconstruction: The Case of the Proto-Athabascan Kinship System* (Cambridge: Cambridge University Press, 1975).

23. E. T. Hall, Jr., "Recent clues to Athapascan prehistory in the Southwest," *American Anthropologist* 46(1944):98–105.

24. Underhill, *The Navajos,* p. 42.

25. A. Hrdlicka, *Physiological and Medical Observations Among the Indians of the Southwestern United States and Northern Mexico,* Bulletin no. 34, Bureau of American Ethnology, Smithsonian Institution (Washington, DC: U.S. Government Printing Office, 1908), p. 8.

26. D. Keur, "A chapter in Navajo–Pueblo relations," *American Antiquity* 10(1944): 75–86.

27. D. F. Aberle, "Navajo exogamic rules and preferred marriages," in L. S. Cordell and S. Beckerman, eds., *The Versatility of Kinship: Essays Presented to Harry W. Basehart* (New York: Academic Press, 1980).

28. R. H. Lowie, *Primitive Society* (New York: Harper Bros., 1961), p. 193.

29. Evidence for the development of conflict between the sexes is discussed in J. E. Levy, R. Neutra, and D. Parker, *Hand Trembling, Frenzy Witchcraft, and Moth Madness: A Study of Navajo Seizure Disorders* (Tucson: University of Arizona Press, 1987).

30. G. Bailey and R. G. Bailey, *A History of the Navajos: The Reservation Years* (Santa Fe: School of American Research Press, 1986), p. 17.

31. R. S. McPherson, "Ricos and Pobres: Wealth distribution on the Navajo Reservation in 1915," *New Mexico Historical Review* 60(1986):415–34; E. Henderson, "Navajo

livestock wealth and the effects of the stock reduction program of the 1930s," *Journal of Anthropological Research* 45(1989):380.

32. Bailey and Bailey, *A History of the Navajos*, p. 180.

33. D. F. Aberle, *The Peyote Religion Among the Navajo* (Chicago: Aldine, 1966).

34. Bailey and Bailey, *A History of the Navajos*, pp. 19–20.

35. D. Johnston, *An Analysis of Sources of Information on the Population of the Navaho*, Bulletin no. 197, Bureau of American Ethnology, Smithsonian Institution (Washington, DC: U.S. Government Printing Office, 1966), pp. 136–38.

36. Snipp, *American Indians*, pp. 87, 328.

37. Palsano et al., *American Indian and Alaska Native Areas*.

38. Johnston, *An Analysis of Sources of Information*, p. 150.

39. "The consumption group is defined as one that constantly and habitually funds and shares all forms of income, including agricultural products, livestock and livestock products, and goods purchased from the traders. The consumption group is, in the majority of instances, identical with the biological family, but it consists frequently of two or more related biological families and occasionally of unrelated biological families or individuals. See Section of Conservation Economics, Statistical Summary, Human Dependency Survey, Navajo and Hopi reservations, Navajo area, Region 8, Soil Conservation Service (Washington, DC: U.S. Department of Agriculture, 1939), on file in the library of the Museum of Northern Arizona, Flagstaff.

40. For example, Aberle, *The Peyote Religion*.

41. Levy et al., "Hopi deviance," p. 387; E. B. Henderson, "Kaibeto Plateau ceremonialists: 1860–1980," in D. M. Brugge and C. J. Frisbie, eds., *Navajo Religion and Culture: Selected Views. Papers in Honor of L. C. Wyman* (Santa Fe: Museum of New Mexico Press, 1982), pp. 164–75.

42. S. J. Kunitz, *Disease Change and the Role of Medicine: The Navajo Experience* (Berkeley and Los Angeles: University of California Press, 1983), p. 32.

43. S. J. Kunitz, "Factors influencing recent Navajo and Hopi population change," *Human Organization* 33(1974):7–16.

44. S. R. Johansson and S. H. Preston, "Tribal demography: The Hopi and Navajo populations as seen through manuscripts from the 1900 U.S. Census," *Social Science History* 3(1978):1–33.

45. D. E. Stannard, "Disease and infertility: A new look at the demographic collapse of native populations in the wake of Western contact," *Journal of American Studies* 24(1990):325–50.

46. Levy, *Orayve Revisited*.

47. The Navajos had far fewer childless women than expected, and the First and Second Mesas had far more: chi square $= 11.15$; $df = 3$; $p = .01$.

48. M. Bradfield, "The changing pattern of Hopi agriculture," Royal Anthropological Institute of Great Britain and Ireland occasional paper no. 30, 1971, p. 62.

49. H. S. Colton, *Black Sand* (Albuquerque: University of New Mexico Press, 1960), pp. 112–13.

50. Ibid., p. 115.

51. M. Titiev, *The Hopi Indians of Old Oraibi: Change and Continuity* (Ann Arbor: University of Michigan Press, 1972), p. 335.

52. M. Titiev, "Old Oraibi, a study of the Hopi Indians of Third Mesa," papers of the Peabody Museum of American Archaeology and Ethnology, Harvard University, vol. 22, no. 1, Cambridge, MA, 1944, p. 31; F. L. Bailey, "Some sex beliefs and practices in a Navaho community," papers of the Peabody Museum of American Archaeology and Ethnology, Harvard University, vol. 40, no. 2, Cambridge, MA, 1950.

53. Quoted in Johnston, *An Analysis of Sources of Information*, p. 74.

54. Levy, *Orayve Revisited.*

55. S. J. Kunitz, "Navajo and Hopi fertility, 1971–1972," *Human Biology* 46(1974): 435–51.

56. S. J. Kunitz and J. C. Slocumb, "The use of surgery to avoid childbearing among Navajo and Hopi Indians," *Human Biology* 48(1976):9–21.

57. J. C. Slocumb, C. L. Odoroff, and S. J. Kunitz, "The use-effectiveness of two contraceptive methods in a Navajo population: The problem of program dropouts," *American Journal of Obstetrics and Gynecology* 122(1975):717–26.

58. J. C. Slocumb, S. J. Kunitz, and C. L. Odoroff, "Complications with use of IUD and oral contraceptives among Navajo women," *Public Health Reports* 92(1979):243–47.

59. S. J. Kunitz and M. Tsianco, "Kinship dependence and contraceptive use in a sample of Navajo women," *Human Biology* 53(1981):439–52. This was a sample of reservation residents. It is likely that women living off the reservation would have had a different pattern of contraceptive use.

60. U.S. Bureau of the Census, Census of Population: 1970, Subject Reports, Final Report PC(2)-1F, *American Indians* (Washington, DC: U.S. Government Printing Office, 1973), p. 152.

61. E. A. Kennard, "Post-war economic changes among the Hopi," in J. Helm, ed., *Essays in Economic Anthropology,* proceedings of the 1965 annual spring meeting of the American Ethnological Society (Seattle: University of Washington Press, 1965), p. 27.

62. Titiev, *The Hopi Indians of Old Oraibi,* p. 337.

63. Ibid.; Kennard, "Post-war economic changes"; Nagata, *Modern Transformations of Moenkopi Pueblo.*

64. Kunitz, *Disease Change,* pp. 17, 83. In 1978 the Hopis were reported to have had a rate of 22.3/1,000 live births. In such a small population with a small number of births, such fluctuations are not unexpected. See B. R. Burkhalter, C. K. Ritenbaugh, and G. G. Harrison, *Trends in Infant Feeding Among Southwest American Indians, 1900–1980* (Tucson: Department of Family and Community Medicine, University of Arizona School of Medicine, 1981), p. 169.

65. S. J. Kunitz, J. E. Levy, C. L. Odoroff, and J. Bollinger, "The epidemiology of alcoholic cirrhosis in two southwestern Indian tribes," *Quarterly Journal of Studies on Alcohol* 32(1971):706–20; Levy et al., "Hopi deviance."

66. Levy et al., "Hopi deviance."

67. Ibid., pp. 380–82.

68. J. E. Levy and S. J. Kunitz, *Indian Drinking: Navajo Practices and Anglo-American Theories* (New York: Wiley, 1974). See also M. Topper, "Navajo 'alcoholism': Drinking, alcohol abuse, and treatment in a changing cultural environment," in L. Bennett and G. Ames, eds., *The American Experience with Alcohol: Contrasting Cultural Perspectives* (New York: Plenum Press, 1985), pp. 227–51.

69. The rate of death due to cirrhosis was higher in areas close to border towns where alcohol was relatively more accessible than it was in remote parts of the reservation. See S. J. Kunitz, J. E. Levy, and M. Everett, *Alcoholic cirrhosis among the Navaho,"* *Quarterly Journal of Studies on Alcohol* 30(1969):672–85.

70. Levy et al., *Hand Trembling,* p. 72.

71. Ibid., p. 74.

72. Ibid., p. 81.

73. Ibid., p. 85.

74. The myth accounting for the taboo tells of the Butterfly People (Navajos) who commit incest in an attempt to avoid marrying the Swallow People (Pueblos). They mated with the closest available relative, that is, a sibling. Today, sibling incest is emphasized, although some Navajos say that marriage into father's clan also causes epilepsy. See Levy

et al., *Hand Trembling,* pp. 46–49, 55–59; also B. Haile, *Love Magic and Butterfly People: The Slim Curlley Version of the Ajilee and Mothway Myths,* ed. C. Luckert (Flagstaff: Museum of Northern Arizona Press, 1978).

75. S. Cornell, "Land, labour and group formation: Blacks and Indians in the United States," *Ethnic and Racial Studies* 13(1990):368–88.

76. The influenza pandemic of 1918 is said to have killed a higher proportion of Navajos than of Hopis who lived in the village of Moenkopi, a daughter village of Oraibi about 50 miles to the west. This is attributed to the fact that the Navajos, who lived in dispersed family groups, did not receive nursing care and food when they fell ill, whereas the Hopis, being near an agency town, did. It appears that the influenza among the Navajos was a common-source epidemic that spread from a major ceremonial that many victims had attended. Under ordinary circumstances, the influenza would not have been expected to take as high a toll as it did. See S. Russell, "The Navajo and the 1918 influenza pandemic," in C. F. Merbs and R. J. Miller, eds., *Health and Disease in the Prehistoric Southwest,* Anthropological Research Papers no. 34, Department of Anthropology, Arizona State University, Tempe, 1985.

77. D. H. Ubelaker, "Patterns of demographic change in the Americas," *Human Biology* 64(1992):361–79.

78. G. Edwards, "Drinking in longitudinal perspective: Career and natural history," *British Journal of Addiction* 79(1984):175.

79. These distinctions are not new. In 1926 F. G. Crookshank wrote:

> The whole history of Occidental Medicine may indeed be almost indifferently pictured as a swaying struggle between Nominalism and Realism, or between Aristotelianism and Platonism, or between the natural followers of Hippocrates and those of Galen; but most faithfully, perhaps, as between Hippocratic Cos and antagonistic Cnidus. At Cos men studied the organism, or *whole individual,* in health and in diseases: At Cnidus, the *part* or organ: the disease: and the type, if not the *name* (italics in original).

F. G. Crookshank, "The relation of history and philosophy to medicine," in C. G. Cumston, *An Introduction to the History of Medicine* (London: Kegan Paul, Trench, Trubner, 1926), p. xxx.

80. E. Goffman, "The moral career of the mental patient," in E. Goffman, *Asylums: Essays on the Social Situation of Mental Patients and Other Inmates* (Garden City, NY: Anchor Books, 1969), p. 127.

81. J. A. Roth, *Timetables: Structuring the Passage of Time in Hospital Treatment and Other Careers* (Indianapolis: Bobbs-Merrill, 1963).

82. F. Davis, *Passage Through Crisis: Polio Victims and Their Families* (Indianapolis: Bobbs-Merrill, 1963).

83. R. A. Scott, *The Making of Blind Men: A Study of Adult Socialization* (New York: Russell Sage Foundation, 1969).

84. E. R. Greenberg, C. G. Chute, T. Stukel, J. A. Baron, D. H. Freeman, J. Yates, and R. Korson, "Social and economic factors in the choice of lung cancer treatment," *New England Journal of Medicine* 318(1988):612–17; B. R. Cassileth, E. J. Lusk, D. Guerry, A. D. Blake, W. P. Walsh, L. Kascius, and D. J. Shultz, "Survival and quality of life among patients receiving unproven as compared with conventional cancer therapy," *New England Journal of Medicine* 324(1991):1180–85.

85. For a somewhat different view of the way people with chronic illnesses learn to conceive of themselves, see R. F. Murphy, *The Body Silent* (New York: Norton, 1990). See also R. F. Murphy, J. Scheer, Y. Murphy, and R. Mack, "Physical disability and social liminality: A study in the rituals of adversity," *Social Science and Medicine* 26(1988):235–42.

6

The Health Consequences of Modernization

The impact of modernization on health has been interpreted in different ways by different investigators. There is no doubt that across much of the world, mortality rates have fallen and life expectancy has improved dramatically over the past century and more. Nor is there any doubt that the whole complex of changes we group under the rubric of modernization—urbanization, the expansion of science and technology, industrialization, the shift from subsistence to cash economies—has been implicated in these improvements.

At the same time, as discussed in Chapter 3, there is no doubt either that these very changes are associated in the minds of many with the deterioration of human relationships, with an increase in stress, and with the destruction of the sense of community that is assumed to have characterized premodern life. These adverse changes—the growth of individualism, alienation, and anomie—are thought by many to be associated with deteriorating health. Although no one denies that the incidence of infectious diseases has been reduced in response to a variety of social changes and interventions, it has been argued that the noninfectious diseases of modernization are the result of dietary excesses, exposure to industrial hazards, a style of life characterized by sedentism and the consumption of various noxious weeds and chemicals, and psychosocial stress.

In essence, there are two positions, both of which assume that modernization has a natural history with inevitable health consequences. One is that modernization leads to improvements in economic well-being, to greater individualism, and to greater health.[1] The other views the process of modernization as leading to a breakdown of community, to industrial pollution, and to a wide variety of untoward health consequences.[2] The adherents of each position agree on many of the changes that have occurred: changes in sources of wealth, in knowledge, and in the organization of families, to list but a few. What differs is their assessment of the costs and benefits of those changes. Measures of health are used to validate the different positions, for what better measure of progress is there than the health and well-being of entire populations? Underlying both positions is the assumption that traditional societies were homogeneous and that the changes brought about by modernization affect everyone equally.

In previous chapters it has been argued that "modernization" is not a unilinear process or a single package. Different indigenous peoples have been affected differently by European contact, depending, for instance, on whether they were placed on reservations or missions or whether they were deprived of their land base and proletarianized. In this chapter we shall expand on the Navajo material presented in the previous chapter to argue that so-called traditional societies were not necessarily homogeneous and that different strata or segments respond differently to social change, with different consequences for health. We shall consider regional, wealth, and gender differences as they influence noninfectious and man-made causes of mortality and morbidity.

REGIONAL DIFFERENCES[3]

When the Navajos were released from captivity in 1868, they returned to a treaty reservation straddling the Arizona–New Mexico border that was much smaller than the territory they had occupied before 1864. Soon they were spilling over the boundaries and moving west and south again. The reservation was expanded several times over the next 60 years until by the 1930s it had reached its present size of about 24,000 square miles.

Over a territory so vast, it was inevitable that there would be considerable ecological and social variability. Among the most important sources of variability was the availability of natural resources, which was greater on the eastern than on the western part of the reservation. Coal, oil, uranium, forests, and water for agriculture all were more plentiful on that part of the reservation in northwestern New Mexico and northeastern Arizona than on those parts farther west in Arizona or to the north in southern Utah. Hence extractive industries and sizable border towns grew more rapidly in the east. These provided sources of wage incomes to some and easily accessible alcohol to all. Moreover, the government administrative center of the reservation at Window Rock was established almost directly on the New Mexico–Arizona border not far from Gallup, New Mexico, and it too became a major center of employment in federal and, ultimately, tribal bureaucracies.

The results of these different patterns of settlement were obvious in the Human Dependency Survey taken in 1936. Consumption groups on the eastern end of the reservation were more involved in commercial agriculture and livestock raising than were groups on the western end. Conversely, in the west, consumption groups tended to be larger; the amount of livestock per capita was greater; and the population was much less dense.

Over the next 30 years the reservation underwent very rapid change. The livestock economy was essentially destroyed by the government program of stock reduction. Many Navajo men joined the armed services during the war, and many other men as well as women moved off the reservation to work in war industries. Soldiers' allotments and migrants' remittances brought more cash to the reservation than ever before. All that ceased when the war ended. Not all the returning workers and soldiers could find jobs, and from a wartime boom the reservation entered a peacetime bust that has never really ended.

Attempts to provide alternative employment opportunities were only partly successful, for plans to help establish small businesses were never fully implemented. Instead the health, education, and welfare systems were expanded, and they provided virtually all the job opportunities that have ever been available. Meanwhile, as noted in the previous chapter, unemployment for the Navajos has remained much higher than for the rest of the United States population.

Though there are exceptions, in general the result of these changes has been that by the 1970s there were still differences between the eastern and western ends of the reservation. In the east a higher proportion of household income was derived from wages than in the west; the educational levels of women and men were higher; a higher proportion of women were working; a higher proportion of families had cars and conveniences such as bathrooms; and median family and per capita income were higher as well. Conversely, in the west, male and female household heads were slightly older (aged 41.8 to 48.5 and 38.9 to 46.4, respectively), a higher proportion of families lived in hogans (the traditional Navajo dwelling); the average household size was larger; and the proportion of income derived from welfare was greater than in the east.

These patterns may be interpreted to mean that people on the eastern end of the reservation were more modern than people on the western end. We would argue that this is not the case. As in the case of Samoans described in Chapter 3, so in this case it is clear that a traditional economic and social system and a religious/healing system do not exist. They were destroyed with the stock reduction program in the late 1930s and 1940s, and in its place has been put a welfare system that prevents outright starvation and destitution but does not encourage economic growth. For example, Table 6-1 is a correlation matrix of selected variables taken from surveys of the Navajo Reservation's population in 1936 and

Table 6–1 Correlation matrix: Socioeconomic variables for Navajo Reservation land management districts, 1936 and 1974 (Spearman's rank-order correlations)

	Peer capita increase, 1936	% income livestock, 1936 (commercial and noncommercial)	% income from wages, 1936	Median per capita income, 1974	% income from welfare, 1974
% income from livestock, 1936	−.58[a]				
% wages, 1936	.59[a]	−.82[b]			
Per capita increase, 1974	.03	−.41	.319		
% welfare	−.68[b]	.67[b]	−.47[a]	−.42	
% wages	.06	−.16	.11	.71[b]	−.47[a]

[a] $p = .05$.
[b] $p = .01$.

Note: Districts 15 and 16 are not included, as there were no data from the 1930s.

Source: S. J. Kunitz, *Disease Change and the Role of Medicine: The Navajo Experience* (Berkeley and Los Angeles: University of California Press, 1983), pp. 37, 52.

1974. The 1936 data come from the same Human Dependency Survey referred to in the previous chapter. The population units are called land management districts (see Figure 6-1), the regions defined by the federal government as part of the stock reduction program of the 1930s. The correlations indicate the following:

1. In 1936 per capita income was highest in those districts where wage work contributed most to income and where livestock (both commercial and noncommercial) contributed least.
2. Also in 1936 the proportions of income derived from livestock and from wages were inversely correlated.
3. Similarly, in 1974 as in 1936, income was highest in those populations where wages contributed most.
4. Most significant for our argument, those populations most dependent on welfare in 1974 lived in the districts where incomes were lowest and where populations had been most dependent on livestock in 1936.

The point we wish to make here is that those places on the Navajo Reservation where dependence on livestock for both cash and subsistence was greatest until the 1930s were those where dependence on welfare was greatest in the 1970s. Moreover, the two are causally associated, for it was the destruction of the livestock economy in the late 1930s and 1940s and the failure to create an adequate wage work economy in its place that has led to high rates of dependence on welfare. This means, further, that those populations dependent on welfare are every bit as involved in the cash economy as are the populations more deeply involved in wage work.

These changes have had important consequences for the traditional religious/healing system, in welfare as much as in wage work populations. The major ceremonies are virtually never performed any longer, and many have become extinct. This is so because in the cash economy there are insufficient resources to pay the large amounts required. In the past when wealthy stockmen were still present, they commanded enough resources and manpower to sponsor such affairs. That is no longer the case.

In addition, as demand has waned and young men no longer have the time or inclination to devote themselves to lengthy apprenticeships, the supply of ceremonialists has diminished. This diminution has been documented for one area on the western end of the reservation. In the early 1900s, there were 20 ceremonialists and an estimated population of 600 people in the region. By the 1930s the number of each had increased, to 43 and 1,254, respectively. The ratio of ceremonialists to population was 1 to 30 in each period. In the 1950s the number of ceremonialists peaked at 48, but the population had almost doubled, and so the ratio was 1 to 50. From then to the 1980s the number of ceremonialists dropped by half and the population had almost doubled again, giving a ratio of 1 to 175. Moreover, the average number of major ceremonies known per practitioner was about 1.7 by those still living in the 1980s, compared with 2.3 known by those who had died.[4]

In addition, the number and type of ceremonies used in the area had changed,

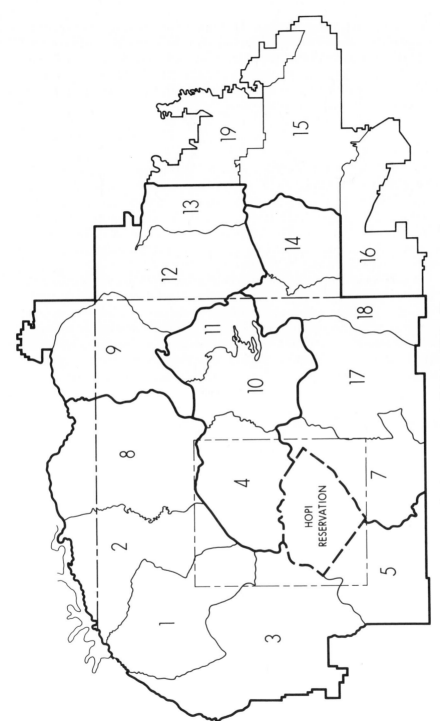

Figure 6-1 Navajo Indian Reservation, land management districts, 1930s–70s.

even in a period as short as a decade. For example, among adults in a large rural kin group, the number of healing ceremonies was 80 in the 5 years from 1956 to 1960, as well as from 1965 to 1969. But in the second period, 62 of them were peyote meetings. "For the vast majority of adults, this did not represent a religious conversion so much as a shift to a cheaper and shorter (one night) healing ceremony that required little cooperation from kinsmen."[5]

In the nearby agency town of Tuba City, the people we interviewed who considered themselves traditionalists had had 20 ceremonies performed in 1956–60 and 19 in 1965–69, but the ceremonies in each period were shorter and less expensive versions of the ceremonies that the rural group had had in the early period. In each case, therefore, the number of ceremonies had remained constant, but the nature of the ceremonies had changed in response to changes in the economy, which had made the full versions of traditional ceremonies prohibitively expensive. Since these data were collected, membership in fundamentalist, nondenominational Christian churches has increased markedly all across the reservation as well as in our study area.

Thus in regard to both economic structures and religious culture and practices, the traditional Navajo world can scarcely be said to exist any longer. And yet there are people who still consider themselves traditional and regions that are thought to contain traditional populations. For the most part, these are individuals and populations for whom a combination of welfare, occasional wage work, crafts, and a small amount of livestock are the major sources of household income, rather than steady employment. Many of these differences are, as we have suggested, the result of different regional histories in respect of the location of natural resources, jobs, population centers, and schools. In addition, the very workings of the reservation economy promotes what Aberle termed "the Navajo style."

> The effects of all these factors promoting under-development in the Navajo country are, at the local level, a particular style of economic and social life—often criticized by Anglos as evidence of backwardness, or praised by some as "the Navajo way." It has some roots in custom, but it has its present causes in current economic conditions and represents an adjustment to them. . . .
>
> The key items that promote the Navajo style are—(1) shortages of material equipment, stemming from a shortage of cash; (2) simple logistic problems in running the household and the subsistence economy, resulting from a need for some wage labor and from difficulties involved in herding, getting water, and hauling fuel; and (3) fluctuating income.[6]

This is not to say that family organization has not changed in response to the massive changes of the last 50 years. Levy and colleagues showed that the various Navajo family structures that anthropologists have described since the 1930s—outfits, land use communities, localized matrilineages, and networks—all have existed under particular historical and ecological conditions.[7] It is not necessary to explicate these patterns here, save to say that the unstructured network pattern in which individuals may call upon a shifting array of kinsmen and neighbors for assistance was, before the stock reduction program, associated with poverty and settlement of an area by a heterogeneous assortment of unrelated kin groups. This pattern has become increasingly prevalent as participation in wage work and the cash economy has increased. Large outfits and land use communities—cooperating groups of kinsmen who are not coresident in the same camps (cluster of related households) that characterized the organization of the families and retainers of wealth stockmen—have virtually ceased to exist as stock reduction, the restriction of grazing areas, and population increase have made cooperation among camps less necessary than in the past.

Thus, differences among populations across the reservation have to do with the different ways in which they have adapted to changes of the past 50 years. In the east, wage work has been relatively more available than it has been in the west, where dependence on welfare has been greater. These differences in turn have resulted in more rapid population growth on the eastern than on the western end of the reservation, due primarily to migration patterns. Young people leave the western end either for jobs in the east or off the reservation entirely. As a result, the western end of the reservation contains an older population that is more dependent on welfare, lives in more straitened circumstances, is more poorly educated, and thus appears more traditional than does the population of the eastern end. (These patterns have been exacerbated on the western end of the reservation by the Bennet Freeze, the result of a long-standing land dispute between the Navajo and Hopi tribes.) In essence, dependence on welfare is no less modern than dependence on wage work; they simply are different ways of being modern.

What, then, have been the consequences for health at the population level of these different forms of modernization? The dependent variables we shall consider are crude mortality rates, neonatal and postneonatal mortality, and deaths due to motor vehicle accidents and alcoholic cirrhosis (for a description of the sources of data and the analytic techniques, see Appendix 6-1).[8] The independent variables we used in analyzing the crude mortality rates are distance from the nearest hospital as a measure of both access to medical care and isolation, since hospitals are located in population centers; population density as a measure of urbanization; and median per capita income as a measure of involvement in the wage economy. Panel A of Table 6-2 shows the results of an analysis using the Poisson assumption and the log-linear model, implicitly weighting for population size. Note that distance and population density are significantly associated with mortality (since the ratio of the estimates to their standard errors is greater than 2), but income is not. The association with distance is negative and, with density, positive. The more isolated the population is, the lower the mortality was found to be, and the more densely settled the population is, the higher the mortality was.

We used the Poisson weighted regression analysis to assess the influence of each land management district, by repeating the regression 18 times, each time leaving out one of the districts. The influence of a land management district is measured by the change in the regression coefficient from the analysis that uses the full complement of districts. In our case, Districts 17 and 19 have a strong

Table 6–2 Multiple regression analyses of crude mortality rates, Navajo
Reservation land management districts, 1972–78

	Estimate	Standard error	Parameter
A. Weighted regression	−3.1653056	0.094152432	1
	−0.0064143910	0.00098212775	Distance
	0.030330302	0.0062701190	Population density
	0.000063166203	0.000094808968	Median per capita income
B. Weighted regression, excluding Districts 17 and 19	−3.2796616	0.13013980	1
	−0.0066342575	0.0013296930	Distance
	0.045790304	0.0067083330	Population density
	0.000026963562	0.00011336575	Median per capita income

influence on the regression coefficients. Panel B of Table 6-2 gives the results of
a weighted multiple regression with those two districts removed. There is a
substantial change in the size of the coefficients, suggesting a stronger relationship between the variables, but no qualitative change in the statistical significance of the relationship.

What this analysis reveals is that crude mortality is highest in the least remote,
most densely settled areas. Differences in age structure do not confound the
analysis, for we note in Appendix 6-1 that according to the 1980 Census, age
structure in broad age groups does not differ markedly among districts. Indeed,
there is a slight tendency for household heads to be younger in the least remote
districts, indicating that the use of crude rates may minimize the differences.
Almost certainly the excess rates in the less remote areas are accounted for by
deaths of young adults in accidents.

The single leading cause of death and the one responsible for more years of life
lost than any other is accidents, particularly motor vehicle accidents. We used the
same independent variables in this analysis as in the previous one. In the full
model, only distance is significantly, and negatively, associated with mortality
from motor vehicle accidents. The less remote a district is from centers of
settlement, the higher the death rate from accidents was found to be. Once again,
Districts 17 and 19 (especially the latter) have an inordinate impact on the
regression. When they are removed, distance remains significant, but density
becomes significant (and positive) as well, because neither District 17 nor 19 is
especially densely settled, though they each are near centers of population. The
fact that mortality is highest near population centers and where density is greatest
is the result of various factors that we cannot measure, including large volumes
of traffic on highways that in the 1970s were poorly designed, and easy access to
alcohol which was implicated in more than 40 percent of fatal accidents in the
early 1970s.[9]

Turning to postneonatal mortality, the independent variables we included are
density; distance; household size as a measure of family size, which could be a

measure of support or competition for resources or of crowding; and the proportion of females and males working full time. In the full model, only household size is significantly and positively associated with infant mortality. The larger the average household is, the higher the postneonatal mortality rate was found to be. The two deviant cases are Districts 16 and 19, with small household size and high postneonatal mortality. When District 19 is removed from the analysis, the model remains unchanged, but the relationship between household size and postneonatal mortality is strengthened. When, however, District 16 is removed, not only is the association between household size and mortality strengthened, but also the associations between mortality and the proportion of both women working (positive) and men working (negative) become significant. That is, the higher the proportion of women working is, the higher the postneonatal mortality rate was found to be, and the higher the proportion of men working is, the lower the rate was. The relationship between the proportion of women working and postneonatal mortality is essentially the result of the very high employment of women in District 12, for in a variety of regressions from which this district is excluded, no relationship is observed.

These results suggest that there is no uniform process at work that can explain postneonatal mortality. Across most of the reservation there is an association with household size, but there are deviant districts where the association is with small household size or with the proportion of employed women. There are, then, three points that need to be explained. First, what accounts for the general association between large households and high mortality? Second, what accounts for the deviant cases (Districts 16 and 19) with small household size and high mortality? And third, what is the relationship, if any, between the employment of women and high postneonatal mortality?

The first question is most readily answered. Numerous studies, both historical and contemporary, have shown an association between number of previous births and infant mortality, as well as between crowding and mortality. If large households reflect a large number of siblings, which seems likely, then both crowding and the effects of previous children—perhaps including relative neglect of the newborn—might be at work.

Why Districts 16 and 19 are deviant is not clear. The conventional wisdom is that Gallup (District 16) is full of pathological behavior: suicides, accidents, drinking, and homicides. Indeed, the rates of all these phenomena are higher there than elsewhere on the reservation, and perhaps that is reflected in child neglect and high infant mortality as well. The highest proportion of employed men is also found there, which explains why this variable becomes significant when District 16 is omitted from the analysis. Indeed, these results reveal that male employment by itself is not necessarily associated with a reduction in infant mortality, although under most circumstances it seems to be. The circumstances in which it is not seem to be those where high rates of social pathologies are also present, for as we shall indicate later, alcohol-related deaths are also most frequent in this area. The explanation for the pattern in District 19 is more obscure. We shall return to a consideration of this region after we have described the distribution of other causes of death.

Finally, what is the relationship between the employment of women and post-neonatal mortality? The clinical impressions of the staff at the Shiprock IHS hospital in District 12 in the early 1970s were that the children of employed mothers were especially likely to be neglected. But a case-control study showed that when neglected children (the cases) were compared with matched controls, there was no difference in the employment status of the mothers.[10] Neglected children (only a few of whom died) were more likely to come from small, single-parent families, however. As in the case of District 16, we can do no more than point to the fact that there is an association at the aggregate level that exists nowhere else on the reservation. Judging by the case-control study, it is not employment as such that is important but some other associated factor that we have not been able to measure.

We used the same independent variables to analyze neonatal mortality. None of them was significant. Even when omitting District 19, the region with the greatest influence on the regression, the model remains insignificant. This contrasts with analyses using unweighted regressions reported elsewhere, in which access to hospitals was associated with reduced neonatal mortality rates.[11]

All the mortality data just described were aggregated by land management districts. Data on alcohol-related deaths are available at higher levels of aggregation, at the service unit level, because they are not frequent enough to be analyzed at the smaller land management district level. Service units are catchment areas used by the Indian Health Service as a way of organizing the provision of personal and public health services on the reservation. Service units generally incorporate two or more land management districts, but the boundaries do not always match perfectly, so one cannot simply add data from the latter and come up with a total for the former. In addition, Navajo service units include some border towns and other off-reservation areas where Navajo (and other Indian) beneficiaries of the Indian-Health Service reside.

Briefly, the data from the 1960s and 1970s on deaths due to alcoholic cirrhosis show that the numbers are much greater than expected in service units that include the border towns and reservation communities that are near them and much lower than expected in remote service units.[12] Likewise, in the 1980s, alcohol-related deaths were overrepresented in the same border areas, most notably in the Gallup Service Unit. In this case the measure used was years of productive life lost per 1,000 population due to alcohol-related conditions.[13]

The service units in which alcohol-related deaths occur at the highest rates are also those containing land management districts where crude and motor vehicle accident deathrates are the highest. These findings certainly support the position that "modernization" is associated with increased mortality from man-made conditions, particularly in this instance from alcohol-related conditions.

The picture is more complicated than this, however, as the analyses of infant mortality suggest. They do not give the impression of uniform changes in vital rates as socioeconomic characteristics change: For example, the more wage work the lower the infant mortality rate. They indicate that there are general processes at work at the same time as deviant cases demand special analysis. For example, the full-time employment of men is generally associated with reduced postneonatal mortality except in District 16, near Gallup. There, wage work is more common than elsewhere, but other measures (alcohol-related deaths, accidents) indicate that domestic turmoil is also common. Hence infant mortality may be high in spite of, not because of, high employment. Again, employment of women appears to be associated with increased postneonatal mortality, but only in one region and then perhaps only as a proxy for some other factors, such as a high proportion of single-parent households.

These results are important because they suggest that in regard to mortality, "modernization" is not a single process. Different combinations of employment and domestic and settlement characteristics produce variations in rates and causes of mortality that can be fully explicated only if one understands the local scene. Thus in the following section we consider the difference that rural and town life has made in the lives—and deaths—of members of two large kin groups.

SOCIAL STATUS

As the Navajos moved south and west toward the Colorado and Little Colorado rivers from the original treaty reservation in the decades after 1868, their livestock grew in numbers. But not all Navajos had the same amount. The great differences in average livestock holdings among land management districts give an impression of homogeneous holdings within the districts. In fact, heterogeneity was more nearly the case until stock reduction in the late 1930s, which had the effect of leveling down the great distinctions in wealth that had developed over the previous 60 to 70 years. The largest stockmen lost the most, the result being, first, that virtually no one could subsist on livestock alone after the early 1940s and, second, that the entire traditional social order was overthrown.[14]

In this section we wish to describe, using the histories of two families from the western end of the reservation, some of the ways in which wealth differentials in the years before the stock reduction program were related to differences in the ways in which young people learned to use alcohol and thus to differences in the health consequences of alcohol use. We consider first the history of an extended kin group that in a previous study we called the Plateau group.[15] They comprised a single, large kin group from the area known as the Kaibito Plateau. This was the best grazing land on the western half of the reservation, and the kin group was led by the second-wealthiest stock owner in the area before the stock reduction program. In the late 1930s he owned over 1,500 sheep. Differences in wealth are not a new phenomenon: The Navajos' subsistence economy underwent several shifts during their history in the Southwest, but by 1850, well over half their subsistence was obtained from stock raising, and differences in wealth had become marked.[16] Pastoralism continued as the major source of subsistence during the reservation period until the stock reduction programs of the 1930s. Differences in wealth persisted during the entire period. In 1915, a survey of the Southern Navajo Reservation reported that 24 percent of families owned no sheep at all, and 42 percent had fewer than 100.[17]

Henderson reconstructed the history of the Kaibito Plateau, which was settled by two groups of Navajos immediately after their release from Fort Sumner and the establishment of the original reservation in 1868.[18] From that time until 1930, the population grew, augmented by immigration from what is now the eastern part of the reservation. Use of the range intensified, and the northern reaches of the plateau were the favorite winter pasture of the wealthy descendants of the original settlers. Differences in livestock holdings increased throughout the period. By 1930, those families with larger flocks tended to travel greater distances between winter and summer locations, and families with smaller flocks had more restricted seasonal movements. The cooperating kin groups of the wealthy were larger than those of the poorer stock owners. Most of the poorer families, perhaps as many as half of all camps, cooperated little with kinsmen who were not resident in the camp. Aberle reviewed the data for family composition and concluded that approximately 53 percent of all family units had been independent nuclear families immediately prior to stock reduction.[19]

The "elite" was composed of families descended from the Fort Sumner period leaders; those of lower status were largely more recent immigrants; those in the middle were from the poorer Fort Sumner period families as well as immigrant families. By the late 1930s, the wealthiest owners, some 7 percent of all owners, held over a third of all livestock in the district, the wealthiest 25 percent owned over two-thirds, and the poorest 50 percent, only 15 percent. It was during these pre–stock reduction years that the majority of the adults in the kin group learned to drink.

Only the wealthy could afford liquor at that time; it was therefore a luxury item that represented wealth and social standing. The leader of the kin group would send a young relative to southern Utah to trade young steers for whiskey. One middle-aged informant told us that the head of the kin group would dole out drinks to the younger men in a tin cup after the whiskey run had been made, and in the evening the leader and his family would drink together in private. As a young man he dreamed of one day being able to afford whiskey and to drink in this manner.

A gallon of whiskey was traded for a steer; thus it was not only costly but also difficult to obtain. In consequence, few could drink to insobriety except on very rare occasions. Because drinking took place within the family and always involved sharing with relatives, drinking behavior was defined and controlled by traditional Navajo values. Cooperation in all family activities and responsibility toward kin were instilled early. The individual strove for material wealth that was shared with relatives. Hospitality, generosity, and care for relatives who were less well off were highly valued. The economic changes that came about after stock reduction in the 1930s were accompanied by a gradual shift to a cash economy and to the improvement of roads which made alcohol increasingly available. Over the years, we can trace the changes in drinking behavior brought about by these developments. After livestock reduction there were no longer any wealthy families, only the poor and the very poor. There was no longer any reason for wealthy families to undertake long seasonal moves. These shifts in residence had been one of the prime means by which families kept in contact over long distances. Families that summered together and cooperated in farming no longer had any economic reason to move to winter pasture where they would cooperate with a different configuration of kin. With smaller flocks there was less need for manpower. Sheep shearing and lambing operations were no longer occasions that required the cooperation of more than a few families. The nature of relations between the wealthy and those of lesser means was altered; there were no longer wealthy owners to whom the poor could turn for herding and construction work. The wealthy not only had lost their ability to sell their surplus in the market; they also had no surplus to redistribute locally through generosity or sponsorship of ceremonials.

Nevertheless, the tradition of responsibility to kin is one that the adults have retained and even passed on to many who were in their teens and 20s in the 1960s, despite the steady erosion of the kin group itself. We note the man who had been a heavy drinker but who tapered off and then stopped after marriage and the assumption of family duties. We note also the man who stopped drinking when after his brother died in an accident, he assumed responsibility for his brother's widow and children. There was also the younger man who returned to the reservation to work when his father died, to take care of his aging mother. Although he did not abstain entirely, he never drank at home and was careful that his pay was not squandered on drink.

After stock reduction, the families that made up the kin group remained near their farms in the southern portion of the district. Even what winter graze they still needed to use was eventually denied them as the population grew and more grazing district lines were drawn. Increasingly, grazing land was in short supply even for the small flocks of a few hundred that some of these families were still able to maintain. The kin group no longer cooperated with the leader's sisters. Herds, in fact, had become so small that there was no longer a compelling need for several camps to cooperate regularly.

By 1960, when we first became acquainted with them, the extended families, or camps, that comprised the kin group had already drifted apart. Nevertheless, four camps constituted a "core" of regularly interacting families, and four other camps cooperated with this "core" on a less regular basis. Together the eight camps included 21 households with a total population of 105, of which 64 were minor children. The eight camps owned a total of 1,890 sheep.[20] This averaged 18 head per capita, well below the amount necessary to support a family. Unearned income from social security and Aid to Families with Dependent Children was a major source of income. None of the younger men had steady wage work, although several worked for a few months each year away from the reservation. The average annual per capita income from all sources was about $360.

There were few economic activities that demanded the cooperation of all, or most, of the camps. Shearing was most often done in a single camp or by two cooperating camps. Similarly, there was no need to pool the flocks of several camps during the lambing season. Gelding horses was the only ranching activity we were able to document that involved men from all the camps. There were still seasonal moves to winter pasture, but these involved single households' leaving the camps to take the flocks a few miles to the north. Transportation was a major problem, however. Only one man owned a truck, and this was used extensively by the four core camps for hauling wood and water and for trips to town, trading post, and hospital. The other four camps relied on help from neighbors and from children who lived off the reservation but who came home on the weekends to help out. Most of the camps worked small dry farms that did not require assistance from outside the extended family. The original fields of the senior man, however, were more extensive and better watered. During planting, five families from four camps stayed by the fields until the job was done. A similar pattern was followed during the harvest which was shared among all the camps that had contributed labor.

Most of the curing ceremonies involved only a single camp, or one camp with the assistance of individuals from another. Because there were three ceremonialists in the kin group, many of the sings were "in-house" affairs, with only a few relatives coming to attend rather than to help out. The only ceremonies that called for hosting large numbers of guests were three Enemy Way sings given by three different camps during the early years of the decade. Each of these events involved six of the eight camps as well as the patient's clan relatives. As we have already noted, between 1956 and 1960, 80 ceremonies were performed for the adults of the eight camps. For the years 1965 to 1969, the total number of ceremonies remained the same, but 62 (77 percent) were peyote meetings.[21]

By the early 1970s, the kin group, which had 21 households in 1960, had shrunk to 11 households grouped into six camps. The decrease in the number of households was due as much to the emigration of younger couples as to death. Among the 47 adults 21 years of age and older in 1967, only six had steady wage work, and seven combined seasonal wage work with stock raising.[22] Twenty-nine (57 percent) thought of themselves as full-time stock raisers. Only five (10 percent) were retired or unemployed, receiving social welfare or social security. By 1973, the number of retired or unemployed had risen to 33 percent, and although the proportion of adults with wage work had not changed, as many women as men had steady employment. Most striking was the growth in the number of women heads of household: from one in 1960 to four in 1973. The younger adults who remained at home were most often divorced mothers with their dependent children. Of the six camps, only one had households headed by active males with wage work. This was also the largest camp, containing three households. Three camps were composed of two households each; three of these households were headed by unemployed women; and three were headed by unemployed men, one of whom had an employed single daughter. The two single-household camps were headed by a widow and by a retired stock raiser who now lived alone with his wife.

The number of sheep per capita had not declined appreciably (from 18 to 16) over the years. Nor did the economic profile of the six camps differ radically from that of the surrounding area. The average annual per capita income for the group ($749) was only $100 less, although purchasing power had declined appreciably because of inflation. The proportion of the total derived from wage work (40 percent) and unearned income (50 percent) was the inverse of the community average.[23] Wealth differences among the camps had become marked, however.

One camp derived 76 percent of its total income from all sources from wage work and had a per capita income of $1,098. In sharp contrast, the camp of a widow and her divorced daughter relied primarily on unearned income and had a per capita income of $491. It is abundantly clear that social security and welfare had become several families' major means of support.

Even in this formerly wealthy set of related families, the disintegration of the kin group was well advanced by the early 1980s. In 1985, there were 10 households grouped into seven camps, only two of which contained more than one household. Five households were headed by men, three of whom were over 65 years of age. Three of the five households headed by women were led by active widows, two of whom had divorced daughters and minor children living with them. Four of the camps were totally dependent on welfare and social security.

Routine cooperation with relatives in other camps is a thing of the past. Anglo-style family reunions celebrating an older person's birthday and Thanksgiving dinners are the only occasions attended by relatives from other camps. These expressions of sentiment, however, are not satisfactory substitutes for the sense of kin solidarity that once provided support and security. Social support provided by kinsmen was predicated on the possession of sizable stockholdings before the stock reduction. Camp size was only one measure of this support, the other being regular cooperation among a number of related camps.

The stock reduction programs destroyed the pastoral economy without providing an alternative means of making a living. It was not until the 1960s that most children in an age cohort were receiving an education preparing them for wage work. But wage work opportunities existed almost exclusively in off-reservation towns or agency towns on the reservation. In consequence, the better-educated, newly formed families most often had to leave their homes to make a living. Today, intercamp cooperation is virtually nonexistent, and multihousehold camps are all too frequently composed of families headed by the unemployed and the part-time employed. The subsistence economy is still, 50 years after the stock reduction, as much dependent on unearned as on earned income.

The drinking patterns displayed by the men and women of the Plateau group developed during the 19th century and were characteristic of the wealthy. Poorer families may have aspired to drink in the same manner but were unable to do so until paved roads, cash income, and inexpensive wine became widely available after 1960. Today, every household in the Plateau group owns its own pickup truck, regardless of the source or amount of income. One or two of the women were able to obtain alcohol and to drink heavily after the loss of a spouse, even though they were entirely dependent on welfare income.

Whether the traditional restraints placed on drinking in the past can survive in the years to come is doubtful. Alcohol is no longer expensive or difficult to obtain. Cooperative, kin-based subsistence activities no longer exist, making it doubtful that traditional values and attitudes can long survive. With jobs scarce in the rural areas, the better educated and more skilled are increasingly forced to seek employment in the growing wage work settlements, if not away from the reservation entirely. Despite the economic and social erosion we have observed over the past 30 years, we have, nevertheless, been impressed by the successful adaptations made by a number of the younger members of the kin group who were either children or teenagers when we first knew them in the 1960s.

Henderson compared the adaptations made to stock reduction by families of differing statuses after stock reduction in the 1930s and concluded that "members of formerly wealthy families have been more likely to achieve educational and occupational success in the wage economy than have members of poorer families."[24] The reason is not entirely clear. Part of the explanation may be that the wealthy stockmen of the 1920s and 1930s, the men who best exemplified traditional Navajo values, were also among the most farsighted and innovative. They were the first to acquire motor vehicles. Several of them used the profits from the sale of livestock to invest in trading posts. Instead of dealing with local traders they would combine their stock into large flocks for trail drives to off-reservation towns.[25] This system collapsed as a result of stock reduction in the 1930s, when cash and credit were no longer available to them. We believe that these men were able to teach, perhaps by example, many of their children and grandchildren to adapt to their changing world in equally innovative ways.

Younger members of the kin group continued this trend in the 1980s. The older children of one couple remained in the home area, but their younger siblings, with more education, completed college. Two brothers work for the Navajo tribe and have relocated to the tribal headquarters in Window Rock. A sister married an Anglo and relocated to a large urban area where she works for a community college. A cousin, after completing college, married an Indian from an eastern tribe who is a professor at a leading university.

The disintegration of the social fabric and the economic decline of the rural pastoralists have not resulted in anomie, a sense of despair, or any noticeable stress due to the conflicting demands of two culturally different "worlds." It was, for example, startling for one of us when a child whom he had known as a 2-year-old from the traditional family of a ceremonialist in the kin group suddenly appeared some 20 years later in one of his university classes as a young adult and an "A" student.

The importance of this story, then, is that it reveals how wealthy families in the hinterland learned about alcohol in a context in which its use was constrained by cost, availability, and the obligations of carrying out a wide variety of tasks for one's kin. Heavy drinking did occur in this setting, as we have shown elsewhere,[26] but abusive drinking was rare, generally ceased by the time men reached their late 30s or 40s, and had few if any discernible long-term health consequences. One young woman died during an episode of heavy drinking, after being struck by a passing car, but virtually all of the people coming to maturity in the 1950s and since have not had difficulties with alcohol and have been successful both educationally and occupationally. This seems to have been the result of growing up in a situation in which—despite severe economic adversity—values of responsibility to kin, the achievement of material well-being, and productive adaptation to changing circumstances were fostered.

The second family we shall describe had an altogether different history, for rather than remaining in the hinterland, they lived nearby and then in the reservation town of Tuba City. First settled by Mormons, Tuba City became the site of the Western Navajo Agency after the area was incorporated into the Navajo Reservation by an executive order in 1900. From the start it was a source of wage work for both Navajos and Hopis. The Navajo settlement became known as South Tuba, to distinguish it from the government "compound" just to the north, which contained the boarding school, offices, and housing for non-Indian employees, with a trading post separating the two areas. By the 1960s, when we originally conducted our research, we wrote:

> In the case of Tuba City, it is not clear that a real community exists in the sense that we think of it in Anglo-American towns of comparable size. The town now contains between 800 and 1000 people. About half of them are Anglos who are employed by various federal agencies. Even though some of these people have lived in the area for more than 20 years, the majority are transients. In general, the Anglos make up several subcommunities depending on the agency that employs them, either the Public Health Service, the Bureau of Indian Affairs, or the Arizona Public School System. The entire Anglo population has little to do with the Indian population, which lives in an area called South Tuba.[27]

The population of South Tuba has always been heterogeneous. The earliest settlers were from the eastern reservation who came specifically for federal employment as range riders and police. Over time, families from almost every part of the western reservation came for jobs, both temporary and permanent. Although some families were related to one another and some maintained ties with relatives in the hinterland, the trend was toward the proliferation of independent nuclear families. Wage work, the zoning of South Tuba into individual lots, and the completion of a federally financed low-cost housing project have increased the trend toward the development of nuclear families.

Wage work has not been the only attraction of Tuba City, however. The availability of state and tribal welfare services and the presence of a hospital have drawn to the area many families that rely on welfare checks and medical care. Finally, towns like Tuba City are, like off-reservation towns, the places where "problem" families no longer able to survive in the home communities must find ways to survive. In all of our research, with Hopis as well as Navajos, we observed that more traditional communities tend to eject deviant families, who must migrate to more acculturated areas. Among the Hopis, as we showed in the previous chapter, the higher prevalence of suicide, homicide, and alcoholic cirrhosis in transitional village and off-reservation towns has often been taken as evidence for the stressful nature of the acculturation process when, in reality, such deviance is generated in all types of communities.[28] For some, transitional communities like South Tuba serve the same function as do the skid rows of America's cities.

South Tuba City has come to be representative of the environments in which increasing numbers of younger Navajos learn about drinking. Growing up in a wage work community like South Tuba is already qualitatively different from growing up in the pastoral hinterlands of the reservation and may represent the future of drinking on the Navajo Reservation more closely than the Plateau. The elements that foster drinking and problem drinking in Tuba City are (1) easier access to sources of alcohol; (2) greater availability of cash; (3) the absence of functioning kin groups and the responsibilities and values they foster; (4) the density of the settlement, which makes it impossible for the drinker to avoid the pressure to drink from his "drinking buddies"; (5) the growing prevalence of the "empty nest" phenomenon among women in nuclear families whose children have grown and left the home; and most important, (6) the absence of a sense of community, making it difficult to foster new attitudes and cooperative activities.

In stark contrast with the plateau, South Tuba was home to several families in which almost all the adults drank heavily and which were virtually destroyed by alcohol abuse. One was an extended family we call, after its eldest male member about whom we have information, the Medicine family.[29]

The man we call Medicine came to Tuba City as a young adult in 1920 or a little earlier. Following a relatively common Navajo pattern, he married two women, one considerably older than he, with whom he had no children, and one much younger, with whom he had 13 children. The older of his two wives had 90 sheep in 1940, and he and his younger wife had 58. Among them they also had about 15 acres of land in an irrigated area not far from Tuba City. In addition, Medicine was also a minor ceremonialist. The family was not wealthy, as the Plateau group was, but neither were they poor, for through the 1940s they combined income from livestock and ceremonialism, as well as from the purchase of alcoholic beverages off reservation for resale on reservation and, it appears, from the sale of home brew Medicine made himself. His bootlegging activities evidently did not lower him in the estimation of others, for by all accounts he was a forceful, active, and respected figure.

In addition to selling alcoholic beverages, he also consumed them. But he virtually never drank at home until he became old and infirm; he was never abusive to his children, though he was said to be strict—sometimes to the point of harshness—with his older sons, and his use of alcohol never interfered with his ability to perform ceremonies or, after World War II, to hold a steady government job.

Until the 1950s Medicine and his family lived a few miles out of town. They moved into town in order to be closer to schools and the hospital, since one of their sons required frequent medical attention. Moreover, Medicine had acquired one of the relatively few government jobs available, and it was convenient for him to live close by. And because he now had a steady source of income that he did not wish to jeopardize, he ceased his bootlegging as well.

The move into town was not accompanied by all the benefits the family had hoped for. As we have already indicated, Tuba City had a heterogeneous population. Not only was the Anglo population heterogeneous, but so was the Navajo, for they came for a variety of reasons from a variety of places on the reservation. The neighborhoods that developed in South Tuba were for the most part made up of unrelated families. Moreover, because of its growing population and the increasing availability of cash, bootlegged alcoholic beverages were readily available there.[30] Alcohol was increasingly available in town, but there was virtually no knowledge of its deleterious effects. For instance, Medicine and his wife are not reported to have tried to educate their children about the dangers of excessive alcohol use; even now when Medicine's children talk about their siblings who died of alcohol abuse, they describe them as "looking fine" even when they were dying of liver failure, were jaundiced, and were bloated with ascites; and several believe that Antabuse rather than alcohol abuse killed their siblings.

Among Medicine's children and their contemporaries, social ties were based on proximity to nonrelatives, and for many such ties became organized around buying, selling, and consuming alcohol. The consequences for this generation were devastating. Of Medicine's 13 children, 10 lived to adulthood. Of those, only the eldest, a daughter who was given to Medicine's own parents to be raised and to help with their care, has no history of alcohol abuse. Three other daughters all have had problems with alcohol, and two died of what appear to have been alcohol-related causes. Of the six sons, all have had serious problems with alcohol, and three died of alcohol-related causes.

Only one son graduated from high school, and he went on for training in a construction trade. None of the others completed high school, although all but the eldest had some schooling. None had any vocational training. Thus their parents' hopes that they would benefit by being able to take advantage of the educational opportunities in town were not realized.

With little or no schooling or vocational training, Medicine's children had to resort to a variety of unskilled and occasional jobs. One son was innovative and for a time earned a reasonable income hauling hay from Colorado to the reservation. Most of his income came from bootlegging, however, and when he was not at home, his children (Medicine's grandchildren) were taught how to sell to customers who came to the house.

Indeed, unlike Medicine's own children, his grandchildren grew up in homes where drinking and its untoward consequences—accidents, neglect, and lack of money—were common. Several managed to escape into a more sober environment, as their aunt, Medicine's eldest child who did not use alcohol, had established a camp outside the town and took in several of her nieces and nephews. She talked frequently to them about the dangers of abusing alcohol, and several benefited from having been raised by her, for they have avoided problems of alcohol abuse. Others have not been so fortunate and have developed serious problems related to alcohol abuse, have married into other families with similar problems, and have borne children (Medicine's great-grandchildren) with either fetal alcohol syndrome or fetal alcohol effect.

There is, of course, much that remains unknown about the sources of alcohol abuse, among Indians as well as non-Indians. The Medicine family's story has been meant to illustrate one of the sources of abusive drinking. There is no evidence that Medicine ever drank in a fashion that impaired his ability to function as either a ceremonialist or a wage worker. His younger wife, the mother of his children, began to drink abusively on occasion in her 60s, to treat her depression after he died. Thus the parents did not provide models of abusive drinking when their children were growing up. Clearly, what had changed from the first to the second generation was the environment in which drinking was learned.

That the contrasting drinking experiences of these two families was not due to a chance selection of examples is suggested by (1) the higher rates of alcohol-related deaths in the more densely populated areas of the reservation already mentioned and (2) the 25-year drinking histories of the groups we first studied in 1966. Only 12.5 percent of the Plateau men were still drinking in 1990, as compared with 42 percent of South Tuba men. Even the men in the Antabuse treatment group were more likely to have kept drinking if they lived in South Tuba (67 percent) than if they came from more isolated areas (25 percent).

We have said that the organization of wealthy families was characterized by cooperation among groups of kinsmen who were not living in the same camp. These were the large outfits that early observers described. The poor, and people like the Medicine family who moved to heterogeneous communities of unrelated people, formed social networks composed of a shifting array of kinsmen and neighbors. For many, such networks were adaptive and supportive. For example, church membership among the people in a border town that we studied functioned in this way.[31] For others the networks that were created were often maladaptive and dysfunctional. This was the case for Medicine's children, who had no parental guidance regarding the dangers of alcohol and who were not embedded in a kin system in which traditional values constrained the use of alcohol.

These two families, then, represent two very different adaptations to the changes in Navajo society over the past 50 years. The differences have their sources in the past, particularly in the place that each family occupied in the traditional social structure. It was this that shaped the contexts in which successive generations learned—or failed to learn—to cope with adversity and to make—or fail to make—satisfactory lives for themselves and for those for whom they are responsible.

GENDER

Not only are there differences among families that are rooted in the past and shape adaptations to the present, but there are differences within families as well. Here we shall consider some of the differences in the domestic roles of men and women that have influenced the way they have responded to the social changes of the past several generations and to the ways in which those responses are associated with the prevalence of hypertension.

The preferred form of postnuptial residence among Navajos has been matrilocality. As stock raising became increasingly important to the Navajo economy during the 18th and 19th centuries, men began to assume greater status because the acquisition and management of flocks and herds became a male-dominated activity, as it is in virtually all pastoral societies.[32] The status of women in such pastoral societies is generally low. On the other hand, the status of Navajo women in a matrilineal society was high, for they had a great deal of decision-making power and independence of action. Thus the shift to pastoralism enhanced the tension already built into a system in which a man was expected to move to his wife's family, far from the support of his own kinsmen, and to take direction from his father-in-law while still carrying responsibilities in his own family of origin. Women, on the other hand, were in a rather more secure position because they had their parents and sisters for support.

The potential difficulty of these arrangements is suggested by the fact that the Navajo pattern of homicide has been for a man to kill his wife and then to commit suicide. Often this occurred in the wife's family's camp, forcing them to abandon it or suffer the consequences of ghost contamination. Thus the act was triply aggressive: against the wife, her kin, and the perpetrator himself.[33] An elderly Navajo man reported that his mother told him when he was a little boy, sometime before the Navajo captivity at the Bosque Redondo: "It's pretty dangerous to have a wife or a husband. Some men, when they have wives, may kill their wives or may get killed by them, and some commit suicide."[34] In such a situation, social changes that gave men an opportunity to be independent might have been experienced as liberating, whereas women taken from their families might have experienced the change as stressful.

In a study of a random sample of Navajo men and women 65 years of age and above living in Districts 1 and 3 (the Tuba City Service Unit on the western end of the reservation), we recorded the presence of diagnosed hypertension. It is a condition that is widely thought to result at least in part from stressful circumstances associated with modernization,[35] and as in the Samoan studies described in Chapter 3, it has often been used as a measure of the degree to which people experiencing social change are having difficulties adapting to their new situation. Some of the results are summarized in Table 6-3.

We used several different variables that are commonly thought to be measures of acculturation. Originally this notion was used to describe whole societies undergoing change, but inevitably it has been applied to individuals as well. Because it is not a single process, we thought it appropriate to use a number of indicators of individual change and their associations with morbidity.

In regard to education, notice that for women, but not for men, there is a significant tendency for hypertensives to have had more years of schooling and to have attended off-reservation boarding schools more than normotensives have done. In addition, hypertensive women were more fluent in English than were normotensive women; there was no such association among the men. There was a significant tendency among men for normotensives to have spent a year or more living off the reservation, but there was no such association among women. When only those who had lived off the reservation were considered, however, there was no association between the number of years away and the risk of hypertension. Similarly, military service was not related to the risk of hypertension among men (not enough women had served in the military to analyze).

We created a scale of social isolation and integration that combined measures of camp organization (neolocal or extended), number of permanent residents, presence of respondents' children in the camp, frequency of visits from nonresident children, and marital status.[36] The scale was then divided into terciles.

Table 6–3 Diagnosed hypertension and sociocultural variables: Navajo women and men ≥65 years of age

	Men		Women	
Variable	Normotensive	Hypertensive	Normotensive	Hypertensive
Education (years)				
0	55	11	94	16
1–8	38	6	18	4
≥9	10	3	7	5
p-value		0.71		0.06
Off-reservation boarding school				
Yes	15	4	11	6
No	82	16	105	5
p-value		0.61		0.03
Off-reservation residence ≥1 year				
Yes	75	10	20	7
No	28	10	98	19
p-value		0.04		0.24
Social isolation/integration				
Low	9	3	11	8
Medium	37	9	77	13
High	53	8	25	4
p-value		0.5		0.015

Among women, but not men, hypertensives were most likely to be found in the most isolated group. Moreover, in a logistic regression, with the social isolation scale and education as the independent variables and hypertension or normotension as the dependent variable, there was a significant interaction effect for women, but not men. That is, for women the effects of low education and low social isolation are multiplicative and reduce the risk of hypertension (by 16-fold) more than does either alone.[37]

One of the most widely accepted measures of acculturation is the degree to which people adhere to their traditional religious beliefs. We might therefore expect that if acculturation is related to the prevalence of hypertension, the most traditional Navajos would have lower rates than anyone else. But when we compared Christians, traditionals, and people with mixed religious affiliations, we could find no significant differences. We also created a scale of religious professional participation based on the number and type of ceremonies that each of our respondents knew,[38] but again there were no differences for either sex.[39]

We also compared the prevalence of hypertension in our sample with the prevalence among Navajo women and men of the same age examined at Many Farms (in District 10) in 1956–62.[40] Among men, the prevalence of hypertension was the same. Among women, there was a significant difference: Those in Tuba City had a substantially higher prevalence rate than did the women at Many Farms a generation earlier. There is much that might explain the difference, but surely one of the most likely explanations is that the position of women was very different, with a higher proportion of educated, relatively more isolated women in the Tuba City sample than in the Many Farms population. This could be accounted for by the difference between the communities, by generational differences, or by both. We believe the generational difference is probably most important. If it is, it suggests that the position of women in Navajo society has changed profoundly over the past 30 years or so, followed by a measurable increase in hypertension. The same sort of change has not been observed among men.

There is consistent evidence that for Navajo women, education and living relatively isolated from kin are risk factors for hypertension, whereas they are not for men. In contrast, having lived off the reservation is associated with a reduced risk of hypertension among men, but not women. Other measures of acculturation are not associated with an increased risk of hypertension for either group. These observations suggest that social change has affected women and men differently because they held different positions in the traditional social structure. Because women were likely to live with their families of origin after marriage and to maintain rights of decision making over their property, they were in a more secure position than men were, who generally moved to their wife's family after marriage and whose own livestock remained in their own families of origin. For men, the opportunity to establish neolocal households and/or to move off the reservation would have been far more liberating than it was for women, particularly if they were able to acquire steady jobs—an outcome that occurs all too infrequently. In fact, it has been observed that when a family has a steady source of wage income, the residence pattern is much more likely to be neolocal than extended.[41] For women, such a change could only have reduced their sense of security. Thus the explanation of the different prevalence rates of hypertension among women and men is to be found in the way that the traditional social structure has shaped their responses to the social changes imposed by Anglo-American society.

CONCLUSION

The concept of acculturation was originally applied to entire societies that changed as they came in contact with other societies. Inevitably it has been applied to individuals as well. In addition, given the colonial context in which most anthropologists work, the notion has generally been applied to "traditional" societies, which are becoming more like the "modern" societies with which they are in contact and/or that have dominated them. The tacit assumption often seems to have been that such societies are essentially homogeneous and that members undergo the acculturational experience more or less simultaneously and experience it similarly. This is probably so in many cases. The examples in this chapter have been chosen to suggest, however, that there are many sources of diversity in traditional societies and that diversity influences the way that social change is experienced and the diseases that develop. Modernization is not a single process or package, either sociologically or epidemiologically. It does not have a natural history that is everywhere the same, not across societies and not within societies.

NOTES

1. L. A. Sagan, *The Health of Nations* (New York: Basic Books, 1987); A. Inkeles and D. H. Smith, *Becoming Modern: Individual Change in Six Developing Countries* (Cambridge, MA: Harvard University Press, 1974).

2. M. N. Cohen, *Health and the Rise of Civilization* (New Haven, CT: Yale University Press, 1989).

3. Much of the material in this section is dealt with in more detail in S. J. Kunitz, *Disease Change and the Role of Medicine: The Navajo Experience* (Berkeley and Los Angeles: University of California Press, 1983), especially a discussion of sources of population and mortality data.

4. E. Henderson, "Kaibito Plateau ceremonialists, 1860–1980," in D. M. Brugge and C. J. Frisbie, eds., *Navajo Religion and Culture: Selected Views. Papers in Honor of Leland C. Wyman* (Santa Fe: Museum of New Mexico Press, 1982), pp. 164–75.

5. J. E. Levy and S. J. Kunitz, *Indian Drinking: Navajo Practices and Anglo-American Theories* (New York: Wiley, 1974), p. 129.

6. D. F. Aberle, "A plan for Navajo economic development," *Toward Economic Development for Native American Communities,* a compendium of papers submitted to the Sub-Committee on Economy in Government of the Joint Economic Committee of the Congress of the United States (Washington, DC: U.S. Government Printing Office, 1969), pp. 243–45. For a useful description of the differences between skilled and unskilled workers that illustrates many of these patterns, see E. Henderson, "Skilled and unskilled blue collar Navajo workers: Occupational diversity in an American Indian tribe," *Social Science Journal* 16(1979):63–80.

7. J. E. Levy, E. B. Henderson, and T. J. Andrews, "The effects of regional variation and temporal changes on matrilineal elements of Navajo social organization," *Journal of Anthropological Research* 45(1989):351–77.

8. The following regression analyses, as well as Appendix 6-1, are from S. J. Kunitz and C. L. Odoroff, "Variability in vital rates on the Navajo Reservation," paper presented at a seminar organized by Garrick Bailey, Temporal and Regional Variability in Navajo Culture, School of American Research, Santa Fe, October 7–11, 1985.

9. In regard to road design, major improvements have been made since the 1970s, reflected in a drop in the death rate from motor vehicle accidents. The information on alcohol involvement in fatal accidents is from P. S. Katz and P. A. May, *Motor Vehicle Accidents on the Navajo Reservation, 1973–1975* (Window Rock, AZ: Navajo Health Authority, 1979). The Indian Health Service estimates that 60 percent of fatal accidents involve alcohol.

10. L. Oakland and R. L. Kane, "The working mother and child neglect on the Navajo Reservation," *Pediatrics* 51(1973):849–53.

11. Kunitz, *Disease Change,* p. 83.

12. S. J. Kunitz, J. E. Levy, and M. Everett, "Alcoholic cirrhosis among the Navaho," *Quarterly Journal of Studies on Alcohol* 30(1969):672–85; Kunitz, *Disease Change,* pp. 103–5.

13. Office of Program Planning, *Health Statistics Report: Alcohol-related Mortal-*

ity/Morbidity and Violence (Window Rock, AZ: Navajo Area Indian Health Service, 1990). Alcohol-related causes of death are alcoholic psychosis, alcohol dependence syndrome, and chronic liver diseases and cirrhosis, specified as alcoholic. Alcohol-related motor vehicle accidents are not included.

14. See, for example, D. F. Aberle, *The Peyote Religion Among the Navajo* (Chicago: Aldine, 1966); G. Bailey and R. G. Bailey, *A History of the Navajos* (Santa Fe: School of American Research Press, 1986); E. Henderson, "Navajo livestock wealth and the effects of the stock reduction program of the 1930s," *Journal of Anthropological Research* 45(1989):379–403.

15. J. E. Levy and S. J. Kunitz, *Indian Drinking: Navajo Practices and Anglo-American Theories* (New York: Wiley, 1974). An extended discussion of the history of this group may be found in S. J. Kunitz and J. E. Levy, *Navajo Aging: The Transition from Family to Institutional Support* (Tucson: University of Arizona Press, 1991), chap. 2.

16. Aberle, *The Peyote Religion,* p. 25.

17. R. W. Young, ed., *The Navajo Year Book: Report no. 7* (Window Rock, AZ: Navajo Agency, 1958), p. 375.

18. E. B. Henderson, "Status and social change among the western Navajo" (Ph.D. diss., University of Arizona, 1985).

19. D. F. Aberle, "Navajo," in D. M. Schneider and K. Gough, eds., *Matrilineal Kinship* (Berkeley and Los Angeles: University of California Press, 1973), p. 187.

20. This includes cattle, each equivalent to four sheep, but not horses, which were not sold or consumed.

21. Levy and Kunitz, *Indian Drinking,* p. 129.

22. Ibid., p. 115.

23. D. G. Callaway, J. E. Levy, and E. B. Henderson, *The Effects of Power Production and Strip Mining on Local Navajo Populations,* Bulletin no. 22, Lake Powell Research Project (Los Angeles: Institute of Geophysics, University of California, 1976), p. 67.

24. Henderson, "Status and social change," p. 251.

25. Ibid., pp. 390–91.

26. Levy and Kunitz, *Indian Drinking.*

27. Ibid., pp. 42–43.

28. J. E. Levy, S. J. Kunitz, and E. B. Henderson, "Hopi deviance in historical and epidemiological perspective," in L. Donald, ed., *Themes in Ethnology and Culture History: Essays in Honor of David F. Aberle* (Berkeley, CA: Folklore Institute, 1987), pp. 355–96.

29. The following discussion is based on material collected as part of a study of the long-term use of alcohol among several samples of individuals on the western end of the reservation, including the Plateau group. Collaborators on the project along with Kunitz and Levy were Tracy Andrews, on whose analysis of the Medicine family most of the following description is based, Chena DuPuy, and Scott Russell. See S. J. Kunitz and J. E. Levy, *Navajo Drinking Careers* (New Haven, CT: Yale University Press, forthcoming).

30. Indians were made citizens and allowed to buy liquor legally in 1956, but Indian tribal governments may prohibit alcohol on their reservations if they wish. The Navajo tribe has so far maintained prohibition, although Navajos can buy liquor legally off the reservation. Prohibition continues to be a subject of contentious debate in many Indian communities, including the Navajo Reservation.

31. Levy and Kunitz, *Indian Drinking,* pp. 130–31.

32. J. E. Levy, R. Neutra, and D. Parker, *Hand Trembling, Frenzy Witchcraft, and Moth Madness: A Study of Navajo Seizure Disorders* (Tucson: University of Arizona Press, 1987), pp. 157–58.

33. J. E. Levy, S. J. Kunitz, and M. Everett, "Navajo criminal homicide," *Southwestern Journal of Anthropology* 25(1969):124–52.

34. W. Dyk, *Son of Old Man Hat: A Navaho Autobiography,* 2nd ed. (Lincoln: University of Nebraska Press, 1966), pp. 47–48.

35. These data are reported more fully in Kunitz and Levy, *Navajo Aging,* chap. 5. We presented evidence there that using diagnoses of hypertension as recorded in the informants' medical record did not result in ascertainment bias. A diagnosis of hypertension was made after several readings over several months of a diastolic blood pressure of at least 90 mm Hg. Thus the prevalence rates in this study are probably lower than would be found in a field study in which only a few measurements just minutes apart are usually made.

36. Ibid., p. 169.

37. Ibid., p. 86.

38. Ibid., pp. 50–51.

39. Ibid., p. 84.

40. Ibid., p. 80. H. S. Fulmer and R. W. Roberts, "Coronary heart disease among the Navajo Indians," *Annals of Internal Medicine* 59(1963):740–64. The criteria for hypertension were the same in each study.

41. Callaway et al., *The Effects of Power Production.*

7

Conclusion

> The modern era has been dominated by the culminating
> belief that the world is a wholly knowable system governed
> by a finite number of universal laws that man can grasp and
> rationally direct for his own benefit. Communism was the
> perverse extreme of this trend. It is my profound conviction
> that we have to release from the sphere of private whim such
> forces as a natural, unique and unrepeatable experience of
> the world . . . and faith in the importance of particular
> measures that do not aspire to be a universal key to
> salvation. We must see the pluralism of the world and not
> blind it by seeking common denominators.
>
> VACLAV HAVEL[1]

The second half of the 19th century in the United States saw a remarkable change in the occupational structure and in what was considered valid professional knowledge. It was then that both medicine and the social sciences assumed their modern forms.[2] Medicine became a different kind of profession than it had been, dominating other providers of care and institutions as it never had before, and the social sciences emerged as entirely new professions devoted to the understanding and control of the problems attendant on the birth of a new urban, industrial, multiethnic, and multiracial civilization. Each occupation developed characteristic modes of causal attribution as part of the process of becoming professions in the modern sense of the term. In essence, explanations became less particularistic and more universal.

With regard to the social sciences, Thomas Haskell suggested that the growing awareness of the interdependent nature of American society created a profound change in ideas of causal attribution. No longer were phenomena caused by the individual actor, the local community, or God. Forces generated by a much larger society, though less remote than the Almighty, acted on individuals and communities.

> The recession of causation and the consequent devitalization of island communities,
> individuals, and personal milieux gave a new concreteness and uniquely modern sa-

lience to the very idea of "society" (or the "polity," or the "economy") as an entity apart from particular people and concrete institutions. By doing so it created a viable field for scientific inquiry. For men struggling to comprehend the changing texture of human affairs in the nineteenth century, "society" was that increasingly important realm of causation located in an intermediate position between two more familiar realms of causal attribution; it stood "behind" personal milieu, now increasingly drained of causal potency, but "in front of" (less remote than) Nature and God, hitherto almost the only plausible loci of remote causal influence.

The ever-denser interweaving of cause and effect within this intermediate realm of causation invited a uniformitarian perception of human affairs without which professional social science is hardly imaginable.[3]

Something similar happened in medicine. Between the end of the Civil War and the end of the century, the growth of physiological and bacteriological research created an enormous change in conceptions of the local origins of disease such as those espoused by Daniel Drake.[4] In regard to the germ theory in particular, several points are important. First, the growing knowledge of contagion combined with an increasing sense of interdependence among previously isolated communities to help discredit the miasmatist conceptions of the local origins of epidemics and to trace them instead to sources outside the community or even the nation.[5]

Second, the germ theory was important because it was the vehicle by which "a new standard for theoretical understanding of disease" was introduced into medicine.[6] Diseases could now be classified by their "causes" rather than their clinical manifestations. Indeed, "cause" itself became redefined. Multiple sufficient causes were no longer considered an adequate explanation of most conditions; the idea of a single necessary cause, without which the disease could not occur, now was introduced for the first time.[7] Diseases were now to be understood at a deep biological level rather than simply described and classified by means of their signs and symptoms.

Third, the idea of necessary causes of specific diseases meant that disease was no longer a local and unique phenomenon; it was now universal. The culture of the organism, not of the patient, was the important determinant of sickness. Although Daniel Drake had acknowledged the existence of such diseases, they were not as significant in his thinking as they became half a century later.

Thus modes of causal attribution changed in both medicine and the social sciences. Causes of human behavior and of sickness were no longer to be explained by local physical or social conditions or by God, but by forces obeying universal biological or social laws. This has led to the acquisition of much valuable knowledge, but the attractiveness of universal explanations has so beguiled us that it has become synonymous with science itself: Such knowledge is what we consider "fundamental." One result has been that local knowledge has been devalued. My book represents an attempt to show how useful such knowledge can be, not simply as a supplement to more highly esteemed ways of understanding and not simply as an adornment for the cultivated dilettante, but as a complementary way of enriching our understanding of the full complexity of diseases in populations.

Even considering a topical area as seemingly restricted as the health of the indigenous peoples of Australia, Canada, Polynesia, and the United States, we see enormous diversity in the influences of colonial and contemporary policy, patterns of economic development and nondevelopment, and social organization and culture. Here I shall review briefly the logic of the organization of my book and some of the lessons I think can be learned.

RÉSUMÉ

This book has been organized around a series of comparative studies at increasingly more refined levels of analysis. Thus once disease ecology has been held roughly constant, one can see more clearly the ways in which colonial policy and political institutions have shaped the affairs of indigenous peoples. And once policy has been held constant, one can see more clearly how culture can make a difference. And once culture has been held constant, one can see how gender and status make a difference. This does not mean, however, that there is necessarily a hierarchy of influences. It is entirely possible, for example, that the social organization of indigenous people had an impact on colonial policy, as may have been the case for Aborigines and Maoris and their relations with the British. Moreover, the significance of each level of analysis is likely to vary depending on the measure of morbidity or mortality to be explained. That is to say, if one were able to put all these independent variables (disease ecology, political institutions, etc.) into a multiple regression, with some measure of health status as the dependent variable, it is not at all clear which would contribute most to the variance explained. That would depend on the dependent variable of interest. All this means that I do not see the possibility of a unifying theory that could explain the interrelationships between these various levels of analysis and a variety of health and disease outcomes.

I do think, however, it is possible to draw useful lessons from the cases I have described. They have to do with the points I raised in Chapter 1: that diseases rarely act as independent forces but are shaped by the contexts in which they occur; that in the 20th century, preventive and curative interventions have had a palpable impact on health status in some instances and that both the successes and failures have been largely institutional and political in origin; that disease differ and that in some instances it is more useful to think about the career of the patient than the natural history of the disease; that modernization is not a single linear process and that the health consequences of social change are mediated by the way people are incorporated into national and international economies, as well as by their own cultural values and social organization; and that it is important to be reflective about one's epistemological assumptions and that when thinking about diseases in populations, the importance of local knowledge should not be underrated.

DISEASES AS INDEPENDENT FORCES

> Give a boy a hammer and all the world is a nail.
>
> MARK TWAIN

In the Past

One of the dangers of seeking universal applications is inappropriate extrapolation from cases that we understand, or think we understand, to cases about which we know little or nothing. Henry Dobyns used this method in his discussions of New World depopulation and called it the principle of uniformitarianism.[8] In regard to the impact of epidemic infectious diseases on New World populations, this has led to inferences such as the following: A group of Indians met in west Texas in the early 1520s, all of whom were blind in one or both eyes, in fact all had been blinded as a result of smallpox, which thus becomes further proof that smallpox must have affected this part of what was to become the American Southwest;[9] the high rates of diabetes among contemporary American Indians are attributable to the historic exposures to viral diseases;[10] there were probably two 16th-century smallpox epidemics that killed many Pueblo Indians, though there is no direct evidence of either;[11] disease-induced infertility was a major determinant of population decline across the Americas;[12] and epidemic disease was a more significant killer of the indigenous population than were the depradations and colonial policies of the invaders.[13] Disease thus becomes a deus ex machina with consequences that are everywhere the same, regardless of the contact situation and the characteristics of the indigenous population.

There is no doubt that epidemic diseases had serious consequences, but as I have shown, not all populations followed the same trajectory throughout the New World. It is plausible, I think, to suggest that there was a range of responses, from the Navajos, Samoans, and Tongans at one end to total extinction at the other, with a variety of intermediate responses, such as the Hopis', as well. I have argued that in general the most devastating contact situations seem to have been associated with dispossession from the land. Not all natives dropped dead whenever they got down wind of a European.

The lesson is that extrapolation from the known to the unknown can be useful for indicating directions in which to look for explanations of population change, but it can also result in the creation of a procrustean bed in which the unknown is forced to conform to what we think we know. This is the problem when models cease to be heuristic devices and become paradigms that discourage the search for, or openness to, anomalies.

In the Present

Just as there were differences in the consequences of the contact experience, so there are differences among indigenous peoples in the contemporary Fourth World. There are, of course, many similarities as well. Significantly, it was an Indian who coined the term Fourth World. It is significant because it is only one of several indications that indigenous peoples themselves increasingly see that they share a community of interests and a commonality of experience that cross national borders. Some other indications:

1. Canadian Indians who have had success in treating alcohol abuse among their own people have been widely hailed by Australian Aborigines as having much to teach them.
2. Conferences on land claims in New Zealand have attracted North American Indians and Australian Aborigines.
3. In all the countries I have described, the indigenous people in general are said by themselves and many others to have preserved ancient wisdom that makes them spiritually richer than people of European origin.
4. There is much travel by indigenous peoples among their different countries to learn from one another's successes and failures in areas such as treaty rights, land rights, health services, and political representation.

There are other similarities as well: most prominently the generally lower economic status and life expectancies and the higher prevalence rates of non-insulin-dependent diabetes mellitus and violent deaths among indigenous than among nonindigenous peoples.

On the other hand, there remains considerable diversity, not simply across national boundaries, but across tribal boundaries within the same nation. The international differences have much to do with the different policies pursued by colonial and contemporary governments and with the differing institutional relations between the indigenous peoples and the nation-states that have engulfed them. The differences between tribes have to do with sociocultural differences (as in the case of Navajos and Hopis), as well as with different kinds of contact experience (as in the case of Indians in the eastern and western United States).

Whether one chooses to emphasize the differences or similarities depends on one's purposes. I have emphasized differences because they contribute so much to our understanding of health status. The lesson I have drawn from these differences is that social structural similarities explain a great deal, particularly in respect of inequalities between indigenous and nonindigenous peoples within the same nation. Such inequalities are not sufficient to explain the differences among indigenous peoples from one nation to another. For that, it is important to understand the policies pursued by colonial and contemporary governments that exacerbate or moderate the health consequences of inequality.

THE INSTITUTIONAL CONTEXT OF CURATIVE AND PREVENTIVE MEASURES

Federalism

The conventional wisdom in respect of federalism is that the division of powers among levels of government is a force for conservatism, because one is likely to attempt to retard changes that another seeks to make. This was James Madison's view in *The Federalist* papers, and it has been the received wisdom ever since. Indeed, people and parties on the left of the political spectrum often favor the centralization of power in federal systems, and those on the right tend to support states' rights. This is not invariably the case, of course. Nor is it invariably the case that major policy changes advocated by the left are implemented as the result of central rather than state government actions. For instance, government health insurance in Canada began in one province and then spread to the other provinces. On the other hand, in Australia when the non-Labor parties have controlled the commonwealth government, they have been able to reverse or weaken national health insurance.[14] The political right may use the powers of the central government just as the left does. Indeed, the attractiveness of federalism to thinkers like Madison is precisely that no party can make radical changes.

In respect of the affairs of indigenous peoples in the federal systems of Australia, Canada, and the United States, the received wisdom does seem to be borne out, for when the expansion of entitlements and the protection of rights have received support, it has been from central rather than state governments. The same has been true of the protection of the civil rights of African Americans. In the 20th century the policies pursued by state governments have been more likely to deprive people of their entitlements and lands than have those of central governments. I am not suggesting that central governments have always been beneficent, however, only that they have been more readily pressured to protect the rights of indigenous peoples than have state governments. Such pressure has for the most part been generated by liberal urban constituencies and is therefore a product of the 20th century, when these three federations all became predominantly urban. This means that what is fundamental is not a centralized federal system per se but urbanization, which produces both political liberalism and constituencies that are not in competition for natural resources.

Another feature of federalism is said to be that state and lower levels of government are more responsive to citizens than are central governments. But surely there is nothing inevitable about this feature of decentralized systems, either. The Queensland government was particularly responsive to international mining consortiums and resort developers, not to its Aboriginal citizens. State governments in the American South were more responsive to their white citizens than to their black citizens. There is no reason to think that one level of government is necessarily more beneficent than another simply because it is "closer" to the people. That depends on the local distribution of power and influence. On the other hand, as the example of government health insurance in Canada demonstrates, there is no reason to think that state governments are necessarily less responsive to the needs of their citizens than are central governments. Gwendolyn Gray wrote that "the institutions of federalism operate in very different social, political, economic and cultural settings."[15] That is, knowing that a government system is federal instead of unitary does not mean one can predict what its policies will be in any particular domain. The lesson is that there is no natural history of federalism, any more than there is of any other social institution.

Universal Entitlements and Categorical Programs

I observed in Chapter 2 that the life expectancy of American Indians is greater than that of Canadian Indians, Maoris, and Aborigines, and I suggested that the availability of a free health care system for many American Indians has contributed substantially to this pattern. That is, in the country without universal entitlement to health care, the mortality of indigenous peoples was lower than in those countries with such entitlements, precisely because the absence of entitlements meant that a comprehensive categorical program exclusively for Indians was created.

This points to an important dilemma in respect of the provision of health and other services. Health care policy in the United States has often been criticized—appropriately, I believe—for using piecemeal categorical programs for specific populations or conditions instead of developing a universal health care system. The American Indian example suggests, however, that categorical programs have much to be said for them, for they may provide services that are particularly responsive to the needs of the special populations that are their beneficiaries. It is not clear that systems of universal entitlement are as likely to do that, particularly in trying economic circumstances or in populations with great disparities in wealth and physical access to services.

Universal entitlement programs can, of course, be responsive to the special needs of particular segments of their population, as exemplified by the health programs for Maoris in New Zealand in the post–World War II period. And categorical programs may be so underfunded as to be of little help to the beneficiaries. In the United States, for instance, categorical programs for poor people—such as Medicaid, which is jointly paid for by the federal and state governments—were sufficiently underfunded in the 1980s that most causes of death amenable to medical interventions were lower for American Indians (beneficiaries of their own program) than for African Americans (many of whom were Medicaid beneficiaries or had no insurance at all).[16] A survey of several racial and ethnic groups indicted that in 1987, 54.9 percent of the American Indians surveyed were uninsured or were beneficiaries of the Indian Health Service (IHS). That is, in this survey, those without insurance (private or public) received services from the IHS. The remainder had private or other forms of public coverage. Virtually all Indians in the survey thus had some form of coverage. In contrast, 12.4 percent of white Americans, 22 percent of African Americans, and 31.5 percent of Hispanics in the survey were uninsured.[17] In that same year, maternal mortality was 7.1 per 100,000 live births for Indians and Alaska natives, 6.6 for all races in the United States, and 12.0 for all races other than white. Infant mortality followed a similar pattern: It was 9.3 per 1,000 lives births among American Indians, 14.6 among Alaska natives, 10.1 among all races, 15.4 for all races other than white, and 17.9 for African Americans. Even if the rate for Indians is an undercount, as some writers believe, it is still substantially lower than the rate among African Americans.[18] Both infant and maternal mortality are considered causes of death amenable to medical intervention.

Indeed, the risk of creating a universal program is that the minimum benefits will be inadequate for those most in need, and those with resources will be able to purchase extra benefits, thus recreating a two-tiered system in which the bottom tier is only marginally better off than it was without a universal system. I am, of course, writing from an American experience. The lesson that I have drawn from the comparison of Indians, Maoris, and Aborigines—that in many circumstances comprehensive programs for particular populations may be of more benefit than a single universal system—reflects my unease with the likely inadequacies of the system of universal entitlements that may be developed in this country. My unease stems from the constraints imposed by an enormous budget deficit, the high costs of buying the cooperation of entrenched interests such as commercial insurance companies and organized medicine, and the unwillingness of the more fortunate strata of society to expend the resources necessary to support a health care system truly responsive to the needs of the least fortunate.

Economic Development and Health Services

There has been a lively debate among historical demographers, as well as among people concerned with health policy, about the relative importance of economic development and health services for improving the health of populations, in both the past and the present. The evidence from the experience of peoples I have described is mixed. There is no doubt that health services can have a great impact: This is the lesson of the American Indian and American Samoan examples. But the lesson of the example of Aborigines is that to be truly effective, health services must be construed broadly. If they are not, if they are focused simply on child survival or if the services are fragmented, then the life expectancy and health of the total population may very well fail to improve.

There is no doubt, either, that economic development, whatever its other costs, may contribute enormously to an improvement in life expectancy. The native Hawaiian experience would seem to indicate that. The other costs in this case refer to dispossession and loss of land, culture, and community, as is true of most of the other people I have considered. These can scarcely be considered trivial, but under certain circumstances, improvements in contemporary life expectancy seem to be separable from them.

The lesson is that health care and social services can make a difference and ought not to be dismissed as a bottomless pit into which money is dropped and from which there is no measurable benefit. Clearly this may be expensive, and many people may believe that for economic, political, and moral reasons that it is not a good way to spend money. But that is not the point. The point is that such services can and do make a difference to the health of their beneficiaries.

This is important. For at least the past 15 years the weight of the argument in population history has been that since medical care made no difference in the 19th century, it also has made none in the 20th.[19] Such a seemingly arcane argument has had far-reaching consequences, for it has provided legitimacy for those wishing to reduce the costs of care, which usually translates into reducing access to care for the poor and near poor. The evidence from the experience of the peoples I have considered suggests that under certain circumstances, accessible care has had a noticeable impact on health, most observable in infant and child as well as maternal mortality. In addition, however, there has been a measurable change in the severity of infectious diseases at all ages, due largely to the increasing availability of antibiotics since the 1940s and not readily reflected in mortality statistics. On the other hand, the impact of medical interventions on the lethality and severity of noninfectious chronic diseases has been much less obvious.

NATURAL HISTORY AND CAREER

> O body swayed to music, O brightening glance,
> How can we know the dancer from the dance?
> W. B. YEATS, "Among Schoolchildren"

One of the consequences of the decline in the acute infectious diseases has been what Walsh McDermott called the loss of physicians' predictive capacity.

> So long as the pattern of illness/disease was so frequently that of an obvious microbial disease among the younger members of the population, the knowledge base on which the physician's ability to forecast rested was reasonably accurate. But the pattern of illness faced by the United States physician today is no longer so much a matter of obvious microbial disease among the young, but of highly diverse hidden structural diseases. With them, there may be one or more decades between actual, undetected onset and outcome. The same basic disease, e.g., coronary heart disease, has many subtly different subsets, each with its own prognosis.
>
> Textbooks of medicine, which can easily communicate the prognosis of pneumonia or rabies with accuracy, can provide only the most general sort of information about such maladies as coronary heart disease, rheumatoid arthritis, or cancer of the prostate that today claim the physician's attention. For although a particular chronic disease may be common, its individual diverse subsets may be sufficiently numerous as to afford a single physician encounters with only one or two examples of each expression in his or her professional lifetime.[20]

McDermott thought that assembling large numbers of cases of the same disease and analyzing them with computers would result in physicians' regaining their lost predictive capacity, and well it might in some instances. This would be a welcome development, for the ability to provide a prognosis is central to the physician's task. A prognosis is much of what we want when we feel poorly and seek a physician's help, and it is knowledge of the natural history of disease that makes it possible.

But what if there is no natural history? What if the trajectory of some conditions is so shaped by the patient's social and cultural context that a prognosis remains impossible, even after large numbers of cases have been assembled, followed, and analyzed? This seems entirely plausible, particularly in those conditions that have been called "I am" diseases:[21] "I am" a schizophrenic, hypertensive, diabetic, alcoholic, cirrhotic, epileptic, and so on. These are conditions in which the patient's self-identity and the disease process become so fused as to shape the course in ways that may not be predictable at the onset, that is, when one can no longer distinguish the sufferer from the disease. It is in such conditions that the notion of career may have some advantages over that of natural history, for it permits us to understand the course as a result of the interaction of the patient with his or her disease on the one hand and the socio-cultural environment on the other. In such conditions, it is difficult to see the disease as an entity independent of the patient. Of course, since social environments are often similar, they may shape disease trajectories similarly as well, making prediction more nearly possible. The examples of cirrhosis and epilepsy among Navajos and Hopis indicate that such consistently different patterns exist and that knowing about them may be useful for predictive purposes. That is to say, knowing the social history of certain diseases may prove more useful than knowing their natural history.

THE HEALTH CONSEQUENCES OF TRADITIONALISM AND MODERNITY

The two theories of modernization that have dominated in the West, Marxism and functionalism, share the assumption that societies unfold in an inevitable fashion. One difficulty with this notion, as a number of writers have insisted, is that the economic and social development that is said to be characteristic of modernization has another side, the lack of development resulting from a society's or community's location at the periphery of the world economy. So the Samoan planters described in Chapter 3 were doing all they could to participate in the world economy, but it was virtually impossible for them to achieve what they wished to achieve. They appeared to be "traditional" and have been so considered, but the reality is more complex than that. Likewise, the wealthiest Navajo families described in Chapter 6 had in the 1920s and 1930s begun to involve themselves in a very sophisticated fashion in the cash economy, several of them competing directly with Anglo-American traders. The destruction of their livestock economy ended this sort of participation, as the Navajos could no longer obtain credit to maintain their trading operations. In both the Samoan and Navajo cases, therefore, people who were highly "traditional" were willing and able to participate in the market economy until external forces marginalized them. Something similar happened among Indians in the fur trade in Canada and among Aborigines working in the pastoral industry in Australia. In the first case, changes in European fashion meant that the industry died. In the second, the granting of award wages made pastoralists unwilling to continue to employ Aboriginal stockmen.

What seems to be true in each of these instances is that the impossibility of economic growth has given traditional modes of behavior a continuing survival value: subsistence farming in Samoa, for instance, and the persistence of extended family networks and the maintenance of even small flocks of sheep as a hedge against unemployment among the Navajos. It is this, I think, that makes many of the peoples I have described appear to be traditional, even though the world they inhabit is very far from being the world conjured up by that term and even though many of them have made substantial efforts to participate in the modern world.

How, then, do traditionalism and modernity influence health and disease? The discussion of the differences between Hopis and Navajos provides part of an answer. In the case of American Indians, it was land rather than labor that was the commodity most desired by Europeans. This led to the establishment of reservations that were smaller than the areas used previously, the provision of services in return for signing treaties, and later the extraction of the natural resources of reservations by non-Indians. The result of all this has been that tribal identities and important elements of local cultures have survived, albeit in much modified form, at the same time that there has been little or no economic growth. Thus differences among tribes have persisted even as they have been integrated into the most peripheral locations of regional and national economies.

With the diminution in acute infectious diseases—largely the result of preventive and curative interventions—the conditions that remain are chronic and often psychosocial in origin. The differences in their incidence, prevalence, and trajectory are largely explained by persisting differences among tribes. This is true of alcohol use as well as motor vehicle accidents and other cause of violent death.[22] As we showed in Chapter 6, however, because these populations have undergone profound changes as well, many of these disease patterns have also changed and will continue to do so in future. Among American Indians, causes of alcohol-related mortality have declined over the past 15 years, at least partly in response to the rapid growth of prevention and treatment programs.[23] These patterns are not fixed for all time, but change depends on political and institutional structures and policies that are not everywhere equally effective, as the example of Queensland suggests.

Not all indigenous peoples live on reservations in remote areas, of course. Many North American Indians, Native Hawaiians, Maoris, and Australian Aborigines are integrated into the national economies of their countries. There are several reasons, among them the fact that reservers may never have been established (as in Hawaii); that people left established reserves, just as many nonindigenous peoples have left rural areas for cities; and that the boundaries of reserves are more or less permeable, depending, for instance, on location in remote areas or near urban areas (remote Australia in contrast with reservations located adjacent to major metropolitan areas in the American Southwest). Whatever the reason, the circumstances and health conditions of these people may most usefully be understood in terms of class, education, and employment characteristics, as I have done when comparing Maoris and Native Hawaiians. Even in these instances, however, the importance of specific cultural factors—dietary patterns, health beliefs and practices, social organization—must remain an empirical question. The case of Samoans in California is an example of the continuing relevance of such factors.

The processes of social and epidemiologic change that occur in microstates and Indian reservations are not likely to be identical to those occurring in the nations of Latin America, Asia, and Africa, though many of them are also at the periphery of the world economy, even if only because they are far larger and far more complex. Nonetheless, there are useful lessons to be learned from my examples: that thinking of modernization and development as a linear process is misleading; that social change may have the paradoxical effect of encouraging the persistence of patterns of social organization, subsistence, and behavior that are thought of as traditional; and that the health consequences of such conditions are themselves not readily predictable but depend on the measures of morbidity and mortality that one chooses to examine and the culture of the people with whom one is concerned.

The Past in the Present

We in the West have commonly used so-called traditional societies as a foil against which to justify or criticize our own societies. Either they were backward and we were progressive, or we were alienated and anomic and they were communal and mutually supportive and caring. Either we knew how to use the land to maximum advantage and they simply occupied it, or we raped Mother Earth and they lived in harmony with her, gaining sustenance from her breast.

I think it is fair to say that since the dawning of the Age of Aquarius, the culturally (if not numerically) dominant view in the West has been to use indigenous peoples as foils with which to criticize our societies' shortcomings.[24] The implication of much that I wrote in earlier chapters is that indigenous peoples should not be treated as anybody's foils. The consequences of doing so are to dehumanize and idealize peoples with histories and cultures as varied as our own and as different from one another as we are from any of them. To lump together all indigenous peoples may lead us to overlook the relevance of peoples' own cultures and values to an understanding of contemporary causes of mortality and morbidity. The examples in Chapters 5 and 6 suggest some of the ways that these influences may be manifested among people who have been able to remain on their own lands, relatively but decreasingly isolated from the surrounding society.

This position is most contentious when self-destructive and antisocial behavior is discussed. There is plentiful evidence that peoples with different patterns of social organization have developed different means of socializing their children and of controlling unwanted behaviors. Sedentary agricultural people such as the Pueblos of the American Southwest have institutionalized mechanisms of social control that have pervasive effects throughout the community and work to minimize levels of violence. Band-level hunter-gathers, on the other hand, seem to deal with interpersonal conflict by means of dispersal. The value placed on individual autonomy means that others are unwilling to intervene to control behavior such as abusive drinking or domestic violence. There is good reason to believe this occurs among Australian Aborigines and certain North American Indians.[25] It is likely that the imposition by Europeans of controls that constrain mobility and force people to live together in unaccustomed ways keep those traditional mechanisms of conflict management from operating and so contribute to high rates of violent death.[26] Nonetheless, to suggest that precontact indigenous life was anything but Edenic and that traditional modes of socialization and social control may contribute to the contemporary problem of violence is to risk being accused of blaming the victims and excusing their oppressors.

This is an important phenomenon. On the one hand, it is a welcome sign that many indigenous people have developed enough self-confidence to confront their oppressors and express the rage they feel at past and present injustices. On the other hand, it can interfere with thinking productively about possible preventive and curative interventions into the endemic violence and alcohol abuse that afflict so many communities.

At another level, it is one more example of the way that we all—Europeans and indigenous peoples alike—recreate our pasts to conform to our present situations. In this case the process has been encouraged by the ecology and holistic health movements in the majority cultures of North America, New Zealand, and Australia. These movements are critical of what they see as dominant in the Western tradition: positivism in science, Cartesianism in medicine, and rapaciousness in respect of the earth's resources. Non-Western people, including but not limited to the indigenous people of these lands, are assumed to have been different and are held up as ideals to be emulated by white Westerners. Whether any or all of them were or were not as ecologically and holistically minded as many think is an empirical question, but in the cultural politics of the Fourth World it is not correct to say so. To do so may be construed as undermining the claims to special status and political support that such idealization implies.[27] It may also be understood as a threat to the identities that people are painfully fashioning for themselves from the traditions and stories that remain.

The lesson is that explanations of present behaviors in terms of persistent features of culture and social organization are fraught with far more than methodological difficulties. There are, as well, ideological and political difficulties. But failure to at least acknowledge the possibility that it is not simply poverty and oppression—real as these may be—but one's own culture that may contribute to some of the problems that confront so many communities may limit the likelihood of growth and positive change.

EPISTEMOLOGY AND EPIDEMIOLOGY[28]

This book is as much about epistemology as epidemiology. My examples are meant to show that mortality and morbidity in populations can be best understood as products of the way people live, and for this both the local history of the population and the natural history of particular diseases are important. Often, indeed, the former may be more important than the latter. Generally, however, we think of science as the establishment of elegantly simple, universal truths. In this sense scientific truths transcend the particularity of time and place. It is irrelevant to the effectiveness of smallpox vaccine whether a society is organized neolocally or patrilocally. Once one can find and vaccinate all susceptible individuals, the spread of the disease will cease. It is in this sense that science may be said to transcend culture. That is, indeed, its great attraction. And on occasion the consequence of a science-based technological intervention are every bit as successful as we hope they will be. The impact of antibiotics on the transformation of infectious diseases beginning in the late 1930s, the great success of the smallpox eradication campaign, and the possibility of preventing and treating iodine-deficiency disorders all are examples.

Such interventions, based on the assumption that science is universal, leap the barriers of national borders and cultural boundaries. Indeed what is so powerfully attractive about this vision of scientific knowledge is precisely its universality: its accessibility to all and its applicability to all. In this sense science is liberating and deeply democratic. Penicillin can cure pneumococcal pneumonia regardless of the moral or financial worth of the patient, no matter what his skin color.

This vision is so seductive because its elegance, its simplicity, and its universality allow us to forget the many ways in which diseases are expressions of particular cultures in particular social and ecological settings. So seductive is it, indeed, that it has become synonymous with science itself. This is a problem, for not all disease conditions are susceptible to explanations based on the idea of a necessary cause, the absence of which always ensures the absence of the particular condition. Many health problems in both rich and poor countries are still best explained by multiple weakly sufficient causes, and may always be, and understanding their incidence, prevalence, and distribution, as well as their prevention and treatment, may require intimate understanding of particular people and settings. This demands a different kind of science, one based upon local knowledge of social organization, cultural beliefs and values, and patterns of behavior, rather than simply universal knowledge of the behavior of viruses and GNP per capita.

It is clear that these different ways of understanding the causal attribution of diseases in populations characterize different professional disciplines. Physicians tend to accept a universalistic notion of attribution. Many demographers, sociologists, and economists tend to take a similar approach, using social or economic measures rather than tubercle bacilli or vitamins as explanatory variables. Anthropologists and historians tend to be more particularistic. These different ways of understanding causation (e.g., "the biomedical model," "the anthropological approach") may—and ideally should—cross-fertilize one another in mutually beneficial ways. Because they are attached to concrete professional interests, however, they are even more likely to be used as ideological weapons with which different groups may bash one another in a fight over whose way of knowing is most "fundamental." But surely what is fundamental depends on what one wants to explain. I have argued that for understanding morbidity and mortality in their full ecological complexity, it is necessary to understand not simply pathophysiological processes and the life cycles of parasites but also the many ways in which human beings live on the land and with one another. That is what is fundamental.

NOTES

1. From a speech by Vaclav Havel to the World Economics Forum, Davos, Switzerland, 1992.

2. This and the following few paragraphs are based on S. J. Kunitz, "Hookworm and pellagra: Exemplary diseases in the New South," *Journal of Health and Social Behavior* 29(1988):139–48.

3. T. Haskell, *The Emergence of Professional Social Science* (Urbana: University of Illinois Press, 1977), p. 43.

4. J. H. Warner, *The Therapeutic Perspective: Medical Practice, Knowledge and Identity in America 1820–1885* (Cambridge, MA: Harvard University Press, 1986).

5. A. J. Marcus, "Disease prevention in America: From a local to a national outlook," *Bulletin of the History of Medicine* 53(1979):184–203.

6. K. C. Carter, "The germ theory, beriberi, and the deficiency theory of disease," *Medical History* 21(1977):136. See also R. Maulitz, "Physician versus bacteriologist: The ideology of science in clinical medicine," in M. J. Vogel and C. E. Rosenberg, eds., *The Therapeutic Revolution* (Philadelphia: University of Pennsylvania Press, 1979), pp. 91–108.

7. K. C. Carter, "Koch's postulates in relation to the work of Jacob Henle and Edwin Klebs," *Medical History* 29(1985):353–74; C. E. Rosenberg, "The therapeutic revolution: Medicine, meaning, and social change in nineteenth-century America," in Vogel and Rosenberg, eds., *The Therapeutic Revolution*, pp. 3–26.

8. H. Dobyns, *Their Number Become Thinned: Native American Population Dynamics in Eastern North America* (Knoxville: University of Tennessee Press, 1983), p. 13.

9. Ibid., p. 12.

10. Ibid., p. 23. Dobyns confused insulin-dependent diabetes with non-insulin dependent diabetes. The latter type accounts for the high prevalence of diabetes among American Indians, as well as Aborigines and Polynesians.

11. S. Upham, "Smallpox and climate in the American Southwest," *American Anthropologist* 88(1986):115–28.

12. D. E. Stannard, "Disease and infertility: A new look at the demographic collapse of native populations in the wake of Western contact," *Journal of American Studies* 24(1990):325–50.

13. Dobyns, *Their Number Become Thinned*, p. 24. For an alternative view, see R. D. Ortiz, "Aboriginal people and imperialism in the Western Hemisphere," *Monthly Review* 44(1992):1–13. For an intermediate position, see W. G. Lovell, "'Heavy shadows and black night': Disease and depopulation in colonial Spanish America," *Annals of the Association of American Geographers* 82(1992):426–43.

14. G. Gray, *Federalism and Health Policy: The Development of Health Systems in Canada and Australia* (Toronto: University of Toronto Press, 1991).

15. Ibid., p. 217.

16. Studies of deaths due to causes amenable and not amenable to medical interventions have become something of a cottage industry. Virtually all are based on the typology first published in D. D. Rutstein, W. Berenberg, T. C. Chalmers, C. G. Child, III, A. P. Fishman, and E. B. Perrin, "Measuring the quality of medical care: A clinical method," *New England Journal of Medicine* 294(1976):582–88. See, for instance, M. Desmeules and R. Semenciw, "The impact of medical care on mortality in Canada, 1959–1988," *Canadian Journal of Public Health* 82(1991):209–11; J. P. Mackenbach, M. H. Bouvier-Colle, and E. Jougla, "'Avoidable' mortality and health services: A review of aggregate data studies," *Journal of Epidemiology and Community Health* 44(1990):106–11.

17. P. Cunningham and C. Schur, "Health care coverage: Findings from the survey of American Indians and Alaska natives," AHCPR pub. no. 91-0027, (Rockville, MD: National Medical Expenditure Survey Research Findings, no. 8, Agency for Health Care Policy and Research, Public Health Service, U.S. Department of Health and Human Services, 1991). The survey of Indians "used an IHS constructed frame of counties with individuals eligible for services provided or supported by the Indian Health Service and living on or near federally recognized reservations or in Alaska" (p. 3).

18. Indian Health Service, *Trends in Indian Health—1991* (Rockville, MD: Public Health Service, U.S. Department of Health and Human Services, 1991). The Indian data are from the reservation states in which the Indian Health Service is responsible for health care.

19. T. McKeown, *The Modern Rise of Population* (New York: Academic Press, 1976); T. McKeown, *The Role of Medicine* (Oxford: Basil Blackwell, 1979). See also S. J. Kunitz, "The personal physician and the decline of mortality," in R. Schofield, D. Reher, and A. Bideau, eds., *The Decline of Mortality in Europe* (Oxford: Oxford University Press, 1991), pp. 248–62.

20. W. McDermott, with D. E. Rogers, "Social ramification of control of microbial disease," *Johns Hopkins Medical Journal* 151(1982):310. I leave for another occasion a consideration of whether, as chaos theory suggests, long-term predictions are difficult, if not impossible, because infinitesimal variations in initial conditions make outcomes increasingly different the more distant they are. This may also account for the ability to provide prognoses of acute conditions but not of chronic conditions with a long duration, sometimes measured in decades.

21. S. E. Estroff, "Identity, disability, and schizophrenia: The problem of chronicity," in S. Lindenbaum and M. Lock, eds., *Knowledge, Power, and Practice: The Anthropology of Medicine and Everyday Life* (Berkeley and Los Angeles: University of California Press, 1993).

22. S. J. Kunitz, *Disease Change and the Role of Medicine: The Navajo Experience* (Berkeley and Los Angeles: University of California Press, 1983), chap. 3.

23. S. J. Kunitz and J. E. Levy, *Navajo Drinking Careers* (New Haven, CT: Yale University Press, forthcoming).

24. See, for instance, P. Knudtson and D. Suzuki, *The Wisdom of the Elders* (Sydney: Allen & Unwin, 1992).

25. M. Brady, "Indigenous and government attempts to control alcohol use among Australian Aborigines," *Contemporary Drug Problems,* Summer 1990, pp. 195–220; D. F. Martin, "Autonomy and relatedness" (Ph.D. diss., Australian National University, 1993); J. S. Savishinsky, "Mobility as an aspect of stress in an arctic community," *American Anthropologist* 73(1971):604–18; J. S. Savishinsky, "The ambiguities of alcohol: Deviance, drinking and meaning in a Canadian Native community," *Anthropologica* 33(1991):81–98; J. E. Levy and S. J. Kunitz, "Indian reservations, anomie, and social pathologies," *Southwestern Journal of Anthropology* 27(1971):97–128; S. J. Kunitz, *Disease Change,* chap. 1.

26. C. Anderson, "Deaths in custody: Kuku-Yalanji and the state," *Social Analysis* 31(1992):1–11.

27. Ecologists and indigenous people may part company when indigenous people support the building of an ecologically incorrect road, sign agreements permitting mining on land to which they hold title, and hunt and fish using modern techniques. See, for instance, C. Anderson, "Aborigines and conservationism: The Daintree–Bloomfield Road," *Australian Journal of Social Issues* 24(1989):214–27.

28. This section is adapted from S. J. Kunitz, "The value of particularism in the study of the cultural, social and behavioural determinants of mortality," in J. Caldwell et al., eds., *What We Know About Health Transition: The Cultural, Social and Behavioral Determinants of Health* (Canberra: Health Transition Centre, Australian National University, 1990), Vol. 1, pp. 92–109.

Appendix 2-1
The Size and Definition of
Indigenous Populations

The definition and enumeration of indigenous people have been major problems for several reasons: (1) As a result of outmarriage, ethnic boundaries become blurred; (2) self-identification as a member of the indigenous population, with or without acceptance by the community as a member, is the definition accepted in many censuses; and (3) locating indigenous people in remote rural areas has often resulted in significant underenumeration. In Australia the working definition of Aboriginal is a person of Aboriginal descent who identifies himself or herself as an Aborigine and is accepted as one. In the 1986 census, 227,000 people identified themselves as Aboriginal, an increase from the low of 60,000 to 70,000 in the 1930s.[1]

In New Zealand in the 1986 census, 404,778 people identified themselves as Maori, about 12 percent of the total population.

> For statistical purposes, all persons of half or more Maori origin have in the past been defined as the Maori population. This differs from the wider definition introduced in the Maori Affairs Amendment Act of 1974. That Act states that "Maori" means a person of the Maori race of New Zealand and includes any descendent of such a person.[2]

For a thoughtful discussion of the enumation and definition of Maoris, see Pool.[3]

In Canada there are two different sources of data for the indigenous population: the Department of Indian and Northern Affairs and the census. The former includes people who are considered registered Indians under the terms of the Indian Act and qualify for a variety of services; the latter includes as well those who consider themselves Indian but who have lost the right to services. A study of the mortality of Indian people on reserves compared the two sources of data for Indian reserves by province for 1981 and found that in general, Statistics Canada (the census) underenumerated the Indians compared with the figures from the Department of Indian and Northern Affairs; the exception was Quebec.[4] Overall, the differences were substantial: Statistics Canada, 154,280 and the Department of Indian and Northern Affairs, 168,529. When nonreserve areas are also considered, the census population of people claiming Indian or Inuit ancestry was considerably larger than the population of registered (also called Status) Indians: In 1981 the latter were 60 percent of the total reported by the census.[5] In

1986 the total number of Status Indians was 374,200.[6] Status Indians are the population used by the sources cited in this chapter.

A similar distinction prevails in the United States. The Indian Health Service (IHS) provides services to Indians and Alaska Natives in 33 states. In 1990 the service population in these 33 reservation states was approximately 1.105 million, as estimated from the census and birth and death records. This is the population for which life expectancy and infant mortality data are provided.[7] Beginning in 1992 the Indian Health Service has analyzed mortality rates for Indians living in counties that are part of its service area, thus eliminating from its analyses a number of counties in the 33 reservation states. It has been possible to reanalyze earlier data for these counties back to 1972. Life expectancies at birth differ from those reported in Table 2-1. For Indian populations in the relevant counties, life expectancy at birth was as follows:[8]

	Males	Females
1972–74	56.3	66.5
1979–81	62.6	72.5
1986–88	67.2	76.2

The figures for 1979–81 are lower than those reported for 1980 for the 33 reservation states in Table 2-2: 67.1 and 75.1 for males and females, respectively. The difference seems to be largely attributable to the fact that the counties in which reservations are located are likely to have poorer populations than those found in non-IHS service counties in the same states, which are urban and where Indians may have a higher life expectancy.

Complicating the analyses further is the problem of misreporting race and ethnicity. There is some evidence that children designated as Indian at birth are often designated as some other race when they die, thus spuriously reducing the infant mortality rate. It has been estimated using nationwide data that after adjustment, the American Indian infant mortality rate in 1983–85 increased from 9.8 to 14.4 per 1,000 live births.[9] It is likely that misreporting would be less in IHS service counties than it would be in the entire country simply because the IHS is more likely to be aware of who is registered as a member of an Indian tribe and who is not. These differences could also contribute to the lower life expectancy of Indians in countries than in the 33 reservation states.

By the mid-1980s, life expectancies for Indians in the counties in which IHS service units are located were slightly higher than the figures reported for Indians in the 33 states in 1980: 67.2 and 76.2 for males and females, respectively, in the counties (1986–88), as compared with 67.1 and 75.1 in the states (1980). Because the lag is short—on the order of 5 to 6 years—between the values reported for the 33 states and those for the counties, because the data for the states go back further, and because more Indians are included in the state than in the county populations, I have elected to use the state data.

The fact that indigenous people are enumerated in different ways in different countries results in some lack of comparability and potential bias. In Australia and New Zealand the count is based on self-definition. In the United States and Canada it is based on the legal entitlement to services. Those who are self-defined as Indians comprise a larger number than the service population: the total would be more nearly equivalent to the Australian and New Zealand definition.

It is not clear how this might bias the results. In both Canada and the United States, people living on reservations, who comprise the bulk of the registered or service population, tend to be found in economically deprived rural areas and are thus likely to be poorer than are nonregistered or nonservice populations. If this is so—and it is not entirely clear that it is—then one might expect the incomes of the former to be lower but their access to services to be as good as or better than that of the latter. These are not simply statistical perturbations but the result of the same kinds of policy decisions that are the subject of this chapter. They are thus less disquieting than might at first seem to be the case.

In each of the four countries the adequacy of the reporting of race and cause of death on death certificates is likely to be highly variable, depending on where the event occurred (e.g., in a rural or urban area). I have found no comparative data that lead me to believe that the reporting of race or cause is significantly less accurate in one country than another. Autopsies are rarely done of American Indians and Aborigines; the same seems to be true of Canadian Indians and Maoris. This is clearly an issue that deserves more empirical investigation than it seems to have received.

In tables showing the ratios of rates of mortality, I have calculated them from the sources cited in the footnotes. The rates for the nonindigenous populations are routinely published in those specialized references for just those comparative purposes and are taken from the standard official sources of vital statistics of each country.

NOTES

1. A. Gray, "Australian Aboriginal families and the health care system," paper delivered at the Health Transition Workshop: Cultural, Social and Behavioural Determinants of Health, What Is the Evidence? (Canberra: Australian National University, May 15–19, 1989).

2. E. W. Pomare and G. de Boer, *Hauora: Maori Standards of Health: A Study of the Years 1970–1984* (Auckland: Medical Research Council of New Zealand, Special Report Series no. 78, 1988), pp. 27–28.

3. D. I. Pool, *The Maori Population of New Zealand 1769–1971* (Auckland: University of Auckland Press, 1977), chap. 3.

4. Y. Mao, H. Morrison, R. Semenciw, and D. Wigle, "Mortality on Canadian Indian reserves, 1977–1982," *Canadian Journal of Public Health* 77(1986):263–68.

5. T. K. Young, J. M. Kaufert, J. K. McKenzie, A. Hawkins, and J. O'Neil, "Excessive burden of end-stage renal disease among Canadian Indians: A national survey," *American Journal of Public Health* 79(1989):756–58.

6. Community Health Services, *Health Status of Canadian Indians and Inuit Update*

1987 (Ottawa: Indian and Northern Health Services, Medical Services Branch, Health and Welfare Canada, 1988).

7. Indian Health Service, *Trends in Indian Health—1989: Tables* (Rockville, MD: Division of Program Statistics, Office of Planning, Evaluation and Legislation, Public Health Service, Department of Health and Human Services, 1989), p. 2.

8. Indian Health Service, *Trends in Indian Health—1992: Tables* (Rockville, MD: Division of Program Statistics, Office of Planning, Evaluation and Legislation, Indian Health Service, Public Health Service, Department of Health and Human Services, February 25, 1992), Table 4.31.

9. R. A. Hahn, J. Mulinare, and S. M. Teutsch, "Inconsistencies in coding of race and ethnicity between birth and death in U.S. infants: A new look at infant mortality, 1983 through 1985," *Journal of the American Medical Association* 267(1992):259–63.

Appendix 3–1

Estimates of Various Polynesian Populations, 1790s to 1980s

Decade	Tongans[a]	Samoans[a] American	Samoans[a] Western	Samoans[a] Total	Maoris[b]	Hawaiians[c]	French Polynesians[d] Tahitians	French Polynesians[d] Marquesans
1790s					110,000	250,000–800,000	15,000–204,000	
1800s								40,000–45,000
1810s								
1820s						145,000	8,600	
1830s				40,000				
1840s	>18,500				80,000–90,000		8,000	19,300
1850s	20,000–30,000			33,900	58,000–65,000	71,000		11,900
1860s	20,000–25,000						7,000	7,411
1870s					47,000–49,000	51,500		6,000
1880s				35,000	43,900	44,200	9,200	5,200
1890s	19,196				42,100	39,500		4,200
1900s	20,019			40,000	50,300	37,600	11,100	3,500
1910s	21,712	7,251	35,404	42,655	52,800	38,500	11,300	3,100
1920s	23,759	8,056			63,000–70,000	41,700	11,700	2,300
1930s	27,700	10,055	52,266	62,321	83,300	50,800	16,700	2,300
1940s	32,862	12,908			98,700	64,300	23,100	2,700
1950s	55,156	20,154	91,833	117,401	137,100	86,000	30,500	3,257
1960s					167,000	102,400	62,000	
1970s					270,035		80,000	
1980s	95,200	32,400	155,000	187,400	279,255	118,251	119,000	5,419

[a] N. McArthur, Island Populations of the Pacific (Canberra: Australian National University Press, 1968); R. Taylor, N. D. Lewis, and S. Levy, "Societies in transition: Mortality patterns in Pacific Island populations," International Journal of Epidemiology 18 (1989):634–46.

[b] D. I. Pool, The Maori Population of New Zealand, 1769–1971 (Auckland: University of Auckland Press, 1977); D. I. Pool, Te Iwi Maori: A New Zealand Population Past, Present, and Projected (Auckland: University of Auckland Press, 1991); E. Pomare and G. de Boer, Hauora: Maori Standards of Health: A Study of the Years 1970–1984 (Auckland: Medical Research Council of New Zealand, Special Report Series no. 78, 1988).

[c] E. C. Nordyke, The Peopling of Hawaii (Honolulu: University of Hawaii Press, 1989); D. E. Stannard, Before the Horror: The Population of Hawai'i on the Eve of Western Contact (Honolulu: Social Science Research Institute, University of Hawaii, 1989).

[d] N. McArthur, Island Populations; E. Vigneron, "The epidemiological transition in an overseas territory: Disease mapping in French Polynesia," Social Science and Medicine 29 (1989):913–22. Institut de la Statistique et des Etudes Economique, 1977, vol. 1, p. 21, for the Marquesas in the 1970s; J.-L. Rallu, "Population of the French overseas territories in the Pacific, past, present and projected," Journal of Pacific History 26 (1991):169–86.

DATA

Population

In order to calculate birth rates and death rates, one must have at least a satisfactory enumeration of the population. Even better, it is desirable to know the age and sex structure of the population. Unfortunately, the Bureau of the Census has never been entirely successful in achieving this goal on the Navajo Reservation. The reasons are several: Many people live in inaccessible areas; enumerators have often been unfamiliar with the reservation and the language; and finding people at home is often a problem. Many of these difficulties have been addressed over the years, but as yet with incomplete success.

If one could assume that undercounting was the same across the reservation, the problem would not be so bad. Unfortunately, this is probably not a valid assumption. It is likely that people in remote areas are overlooked more than people in accessible areas, and young, highly mobile men may be especially likely to be missed. In our study of elderly people in Districts 1 and 3, we estimated that the 1980 census underenumerated that age group by between 10 and 15 percent.[1] For the analyses presented in Chapter 6, we estimated that the resident population on the Navajo Reservation in 1975—the midpoint of the years for which we have mortality data—was 130,000.

Because we are comparing crude rates of death across land management districts, it is important to point out that age distributions in broad categories do not differ, even though the average ages of household heads are found to differ somewhat among districts, as reported in Chapter 6. About 50 percent of the population of each district was in the 0 to 17 age group; 45 percent in the 18 to 64 age group; and 5 percent in the 65 and above age group.

Independent Variables

We used two sources of independent variables: estimates of the population density of each land management district as provided by the Bureau of Indian Affairs[2] and an economic survey done by sampling populations in all land management districts.[3] In addition, we calculated the distance of each land management district from the nearest hospital (by the most direct paved road from the center of the district). The values of the variables may be found in a previous publication.[4]

Population density was included as a proxy for urbanization. The other independent variables are (1) median per capita income, (2) median family income, (3) proportion of women and of men working more than 50 weeks in a year, (4) average household size, (5) average educational attainment of male and female heads of households, and (6) proportion of income from wages and from welfare.

The source of these variables is a survey of a random sample of each land management district carried out in 1974. The unit sampled was the household rather than the camp, as is the case with most censuses and surveys. To the extent that child care and economic resources are shared beyond the household level, these data are likely to distort the true state of affairs. The survey was based on a cluster sample, choosing primary sampling points in the chapter house area in each district and identifying the points on a map for each interviewer. Each interviewer was instructed to obtain a "cluster" of interviews in his or her designated area. Presumably this procedure would be subject to the same problems of nonresponse as reported by the census, except that the supervision of interviewers may have been more rigorous.

Snedecor and Cochrane give some guidance as to the effects on simple linear regression of errors in measuring the causal variables.[5] Such measurement errors tend to lead to an underestimation of the size of the regression effects. In our case, we have no protection against the possibility that some of the causal variables may not enter into the model because of underestimation of the regression coefficients due to bias in measuring the causal variables. The bias due to errors in measurement may, however, be overwhelmed by bias introduced by variables not included in the analysis because they cannot (or have not) been measured at all.

Dependent Variables

The source of data on Navajo deaths is a computer file of death certificates provided by the Indian Health Service. It is important to describe briefly the origin of this file so as to make clear the numerous sources of possible error. Death certificates are filled out by an attending professional: a physician or a nonphysician coroner. These are filed with the health department of the state in which the individual died. In addition, if the individual's place of residence was in a different state, a copy of the certificate is sent to the health department of the state of residence. The certificates are transferred to computer files and sent to the National Center for Health Statistics in Washington. From this tape, a file of Indian deaths is prepared and sent to the Indian Health Service. From that file of all Indian deaths, a file was prepared for us listing deaths of Indians in 1972–78 whose place of residence had been a community on the Navajo Reservation. It is important to note that the community of residence is coded, but not tribal membership. Instead, race (white, black, Indian, etc.) is coded. It is assumed that an Indian whose address is a community on the Navajo Reservation is in fact a Navajo. This assumption is undoubtedly wrong some of the time, as Indians of other tribes may live there as government employees, spouses of Navajos, or for some other reason. Moreover, not all communities are coded accurately, so assigning a community to a land management district is sometimes problematic.[6] Despite these difficulties, death certificates are the only source of data on mortality that are reasonably complete.

There are several things one wants to know about deaths: number by age, sex, cause(s), race, and place of residence. Death certificates should provide all of this. We are not aware of any studies on the Navajo Reservation that deal with the adequacy of reporting. Our study of elderly people suggested that the fact of death was accurately recorded.[7] Race was recorded accurately on the death certificates, but on some occasions, errors in key punching led to misclassification on the computer file. Age and sex were recorded accurately, as was place of residence. Age, sex, and place of residence were accurately recorded as well.

On the other hand, diagnoses pose problems, as they do everywhere. Autopsies of Indian Health Service beneficiaries are rare. Patients who die in hospital may be adequately diagnosed, nonetheless, because of thorough antemortem work-ups. But except for motor vehicle accident victims, people dying out of hospital seem to be diagnosed in a somewhat cursory fashion—often as cardiac arrest, cardiorespiratory failure, or simply as dead on arrival. We are now much less willing than previously to trust the diagnoses on the certificates and believe that the distinctions previously reported among regions in regard to patterns of cause are probably not as accurate as we had originally thought, though the broad distinctions are still valid, with a few exceptions.[8] Automobile accidents are accurately recorded because fatal accidents come to the attention of the police. Similarly, homicides and other violent deaths are probably adequately reflected in the statistics, with the possible exception of deaths from neglect. But complex, multiple-cause deaths, which are increasingly common as chronic noninfectious diseases become more frequent, are probably not adequately reflected in the statistics. Infant deaths seem especially likely to be accurately recorded, since public health nurses and Community Health Representatives often follow children at home during the first year of life, particularly if they are living in high-risk situations. Neonatal deaths occurring in hospital are almost certainly accurately recorded.

Birth certificates are treated in the same fashion as death certificates, passing through multiple stages before ending up in a usable file. For this reason, we have used hospital records rather than birth certificates as the source of data on fertility. There are several reasons that they are preferable. These records are created in the following way: Each admission to either an Indian Health Service or a contract hospital is recorded on a short form at the time of discharge. These are then transferred to a computer file that includes all the data on the original sheet: tribal membership, age of patient, community of residence, type of procedure done, diagnoses, and so on. Not included are some important data that are found on birth certificates: education of parents, occupation, birth weight, and parity, among others. Because we are concerned here only with births as the denominator for the infant mortality rate, we have elected to sacrifice range of information for accuracy, since more than 95 percent of Navajos are now born in hospitals and since both IHS and contract facilities accurately record tribal membership. If women deliver in non-IHS hospitals that are paid by some other third party, they are lost to the system we have used. A check of records in hospitals in communities bordering the reservation in the early 1970s showed this to be an insignificant problem. Since the data in Chapter 6 are from the 1970s, we have not attempted to estimate the loss to the record system. As third-party insurance coverage increases with increasing wage work, however, the problem could become significant.

Average annual death rates are calculated using as a denominator the population figures just described, and as a numerator the total number of deaths occurring in 1972–78 divided by 7 (the number of years). Infant, neonatal, and postneonatal mortality rates are calculated using the number of births as the denominator.

METHODS

In analyzing regional variations in mortality, we wish to assess the associations between response variables such as crude death rates, rates of death from motor vehicle accidents, and neonatal and postneonatal death rates, and independent variables such as population density, distance from hospital, and income. It is not likely that simple associations between the possible causal variables and the response variables measured in the aggregate can give anything more than an indication of relationships. Errors in measuring a variable, sampling errors, and problems of nonresponse and aggregation all tend to cloud the interpretation. We also confront the problem of committing the ecological fallacy: inferring causal relationships at the individual level from aggregate data. On the other hand, a simple description of the data together with information from other sources may give guidance for further investigations. Moreover, in regard to the ecological fallacy, it has been suggested that such analyses are useful inasmuch as they reveal features of the social system that may be correlated. A high correlation between arrest rates and divorces does not necessarily mean that divorcees are likely to be arrested but is more likely to be used to support the argument that "both arrests and divorces are functions of a common underlying cause inherent not in the individuals as such but in inter-individual differences and relationships—'properties of the area as such'—termed culture conflict, social disorganization, or what have you."[9]

We used a modified form of multiple linear regression as a descriptive tool to assess the relationships between the causal and response variables. We adopted two innovations that have not been used widely to analyze vital rates: (1) weighted regression to adjust for differences in sizes of the land management district populations and (2) techniques to assess whether an individual land management district has a large influence on the regression analysis.

In regard to the use of weighted regressions, the ratio between the largest and smallest land management district populations is about 5 to 1. Arguably, therefore, each district should not get equal weight, and we thus adopted a weighted form of regression analysis to aid description. We assumed that the counts have a Poisson distribution with the mean proportional to the population size in the land management district and that the causal variables are related to the response variable through a log-linear model. The Poisson distribution is applicable to count data when the rate of occurrence is very small (e.g., death rates) and the population size is large. Many vital rates obey the Poisson probability law in practice. The log-linear model is convenient, for we can then use techniques for fitting generalized linear models available through GLIM.[10] Regression coefficients and their approximate standard errors can be used to assess the strength of association. When the ratio of the estimate of the coefficient to the standard error is 2 or more, the association is significant at 0.05 or less.

There are drawbacks to these models. The Poisson–log-linear models are difficult to interpret because the natural scale of the model is the logarithm of the rates. Therefore we must rely heavily on the estimates of the regression coefficients and their standard errors for interpretation. The only real defense we can offer for this analysis is that it leads to plausible conclusions. There is nothing in theory to suggest that the regression of rates in the linear scale is any more plausible.[11] Perhaps the analyses in Chapter 6 will encourage others to try a different set of reasonable models in order to assess whether our analyses are sensitive to assumptions.

The availability of GLIM as a statistical tool allows us to make an internal assessment of the influence of each land management district on the regression analysis. This allows us to group land management districts into possibly homogeneous clusters and represents an innovation in analysis.

NOTES

1. S. J. Kunitz and J. E. Levy, *Navajo Aging: From Family to Institutional Support* (Tucson: University of Arizona Press, 1991).

2. J. M. Goodman, *The Navajo Atlas* (Norman: University of Oklahoma Press, 1982), p. 70.

3. M. J. Wistisen, R. J. Parsons, and A. Larsen, *A Study to Identify Potentially Feasible Small Businesses for the Navajo Nation* (Provo, UT: Center for Business and Economic Research, Survey Research Center, Brigham Young University, 1975).

4. S. J. Kunitz, *Disease Change and the Role of Medicine: The Navajo Experience* (Berkeley and Los Angeles: University of California Press, 1983), p. 52.

5. G. W. Snedecor and W. G. Cochran, *Statistical Methods,* 7th ed. (Ames: Iowa State University Press, 1980), pp. 171–72, 380–83.

6. For more data on death certificates, see Kunitz, *Disease Change,* p. 192.

7. Kunitz and Levy, *Navajo Aging,* pp. 106–8.

8. Kunitz, *Disease Change,* p. 113.

9. On the ecological fallacy, the classic article is by W. S. Robinson, "Ecological correlations and the behavior of individuals," *American Sociological Review* 15(1950): 351–57. The quotation is from H. Menzel, "Comment on Robinson's 'Ecological correlations and the behavior of individuals,'" *American Sociological Review* 15(1950):674.

10. R. J. Baker and J. A. Nelder, *The GLIM System,* release 3 (Oxford: Numerical Algorithm Group, 1978).

11. P. Diehr, "Small area statistics: Large statistical problems," *American Journal of Public Health* 74(1984):313–14.

Index